Text and Atlas
Slit Lamp Biomicroscopy
for Assessment in
Cataract Surgery

Text and Atlas
Slit Lamp Biomicroscopy for Assessment in Cataract Surgery

Navneet Toshniwal MBBS MS
Ophthalmologist
Consultant and Director
Navneet Hospital
Solapur, Maharashtra, India

Foreword
TP Lahane

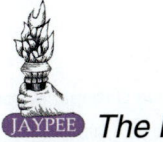

JAYPEE *The Health Sciences Publishers*
New Delhi | London | Philadelphia | Panama

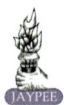 **Jaypee Brothers Medical Publishers (P) Ltd.**

Headquarters
Jaypee Brothers Medical Publishers (P) Ltd.
4838/24, Ansari Road, Daryaganj
New Delhi 110 002, India
Phone: +91-11-43574357
Fax: +91-11-43574314
E-mail: jaypee@jaypeebrothers.com

Overseas Offices

J.P. Medical Ltd.
83, Victoria Street, London
SW1H 0HW (UK)
Phone: +44-20 3170 8910
Fax: +44(0)20 3008 6180
E-mail: info@jpmedpub.com

Jaypee-Highlights Medical Publishers Inc.
City of Knowledge, Bld. 237, Clayton
Panama City, Panama
Phone: +1 507-301-0496
Fax: +1 507-301-0499
E-mail: cservice@jphmedical.com

Jaypee Medical Inc.
The Bourse
111, South Independence Mall East
Suite 835, Philadelphia, PA 19106, USA
Phone: +1 267-519-9789
E-mail: jpmed.us@gmail.com

Jaypee Brothers Medical Publishers (P) Ltd.
17/1-B, Babar Road, Block-B, Shaymali
Mohammadpur, Dhaka-1207
Bangladesh
Mobile: +08801912003485
E-mail: jaypeedhaka@gmail.com

Jaypee Brothers Medical Publishers (P) Ltd.
Bhotahity, Kathmandu, Nepal
Phone: +977-9741283608
E-mail: kathmandu@jaypeebrothers.com

Website: www.jaypeebrothers.com
Website: www.jaypeedigital.com

© 2014, Jaypee Brothers Medical Publishers

The views and opinions expressed in this book are solely those of the original contributor(s)/author(s) and do not necessarily represent those of editor(s) of the book.

All rights reserved. No part of this publication may be reproduced, stored or transmitted in any form or by any means, electronic, mechanical, photocopying, recording or otherwise, without the prior permission in writing of the publishers.

All brand names and product names used in this book are trade names, service marks, trademarks or registered trademarks of their respective owners. The publisher is not associated with any product or vendor mentioned in this book.

Medical knowledge and practice change constantly. This book is designed to provide accurate, authoritative information about the subject matter in question. However, readers are advised to check the most current information available on procedures included and check information from the manufacturer of each product to be administered, to verify the recommended dose, formula, method and duration of administration, adverse effects and contraindications. It is the responsibility of the practitioner to take all appropriate safety precautions. Neither the publisher nor the author(s)/editor(s) assume any liability for any injury and/or damage to persons or property arising from or related to use of material in this book.

This book is sold on the understanding that the publisher is not engaged in providing professional medical services. If such advice or services are required, the services of a competent medical professional should be sought.

Every effort has been made where necessary to contact holders of copyright to obtain permission to reproduce copyright material. If any have been inadvertently overlooked, the publisher will be pleased to make the necessary arrangements at the first opportunity.

Inquiries for bulk sales may be solicited at: jaypee@jaypeebrothers.com

Text and Atlas—Slit Lamp Biomicroscopy for Assessment in Cataract Surgery

First Edition: **2014**

ISBN: 978-93-5152-384-0

Printed at: Samrat Offset Pvt. Ltd.

Dedicated to

*My respected teacher Dr Madhusudan V Albal
who was my guide and postgraduate teacher at
Dr VM Medical College, Solapur, Maharashtra, India*

Foreword

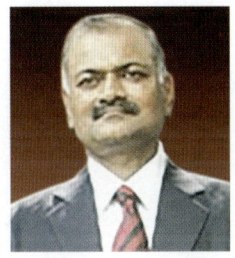

It is a matter of immense pride and pleasure for me to write a foreword for the book '*Text and Atlas— Slit Lamp Biomicroscopy for Assessment in Cataract Surgery*' by Dr Navneet Toshniwal.

Dr Navneet is one of the most eminent ophthalmologists of Maharashtra, India with an academic inclination. Having worked relentlessly in the field of ophthalmology for over a decade now, Dr Navneet has always strived to pass his wisdom and knowledge to upcoming and aspiring ophthalmologists through variety of measures, this book being his second such endeavor towards this direction.

Hellen Keller once famously said 'The most pathetic person in the world is someone who has sight but no vision.' This is very true when it comes to pre-operative preparation of a patient being planned for cataract surgery. Though there have been state-of-the-art advances in the evolution and technique of cataract surgery, absence of careful examination and assessment of cataract on the slit lamp can lead to troublesome intraoperative complications. Careful preoperative slit lamp examination of cataract still remains the gold standard 'insurance' to avoid intraoperative surprises and vision-threatening complications.

Though there are numerous textbooks and treatises on cataract assessment, there was long-felt need for a practical handbook that would delve extensively into the varied aspects of slit lamp examination techniques prior to cataract surgery; yet at the same time remain concise, lucid and illustrative. Dr Navneet has successfully attempted to fill this gap by coming out with his masterpiece. The language is simple, to-the-point with beautifully crafted self-illustrative images that deliver the message intended, crisply. This book is a reflection of his thorough understanding of the subject and outcome of his experience on this aspect.

I am sure the book will prove useful not only to consulting ophthalmologists in their everyday practice but also to postgraduate students pursuing ophthalmology. It is not meant to be the ultimate bible, but be a ready reckoner for a quick brush-up on the important preoperative aspects before cataract surgery, that is important for every ophthalmic surgeon.

I wish Dr Navneet all the very best in his endeavor!

TP Lahane
Ophthalmologist
Honored Padmashree in 2008
Dean, Grant Medical College and Sir JJ Group of Hospitals
Mumbai, Maharashtra, India

Preface

My first book on Phaco surgery *Simplified Phacoemulsification* was a real motivation for me to write another book concerned with cataract surgery. In my mind there were three-to-four topics but I have selected very important and day-to-day needed practical topic which is concerned with selection of patient and analysis of the steps of Phaco surgery, small incision cataract surgery (SICS) or extracapsular cataract extraction (ECCE) before start of surgery by slit lamp examination.

In January 2010, I have been invited as a guest speaker for regional conference of Cataract and Refractive Society of Cairo, Egypt. It was great opportunity for me to visit Egypt for the second time. During that period, one of the local groups of doctors from Damait and Almansura were wishing to talk on Phaco surgery on one evening. I decided to talk on this very basic topic, how to select patients by slit lamp examination. It is just not selection but also to analyze or clinically correlate anatomy of the lens with steps of surgery. This simple topic was very well-appreciated by doctors from Egypt. This was another motivation for me to share such practical knowledge with my colleagues in the form of a book.

Examination of patients of cataract in predilated and postdilated pupil by torch light and slit lamp is very important. In every case silt lamp is the most important tool to see the patient in detail. This will help to see the cases in Gross view, Slit view and Retroillumination. Gross view will give overall idea about anatomy and size of the eye, conjunctiva, cornea, anterior chamber, iris, pupil, pupillary reaction, and stage of cataract. Slit view will be helpful to see layers of every structure in oblique illumination. Most important in this examination is status of the cornea, anterior chamber depth, details of iris, pupil, curvature of anterior capsule, all layers of the lens means anterior capsule, cortex, epinucleus, nucleus, and posterior capsule.

According to me, everyone should concentrate for density and size of the nucleus and its correlation with the pupil size. This examination will definitely give assessment of anatomy of the nucleus which is emulsified in Phaco surgery through a small incision. Setting of parameters on machine, and surgical technique is depending on this unique examination and analysis.

We are in a habit of slit lamp examination of patients on slit lamp from our undergraduate and postgraduate days. Approach to see the cases on slit lamp is different when surgeons really start their own practice. Being a teaching institute in cataract, every case is analyzed in detail before surgery which has been recorded.

This unique collection of slit lamp photographs of cataract of our institute from the last six years were organized in a book. Due to teaching process, everyday I learn new points out of this slit lamp examination, which means "Teaching is the best learning process".

In this book, slit lamp photography of all varieties of cataract related to anatomy, etiology and associated condition are described.

The book will be helpful to all doctors of undergraduate, postgraduate level, for surgeons who started cataract surgery and for those who are already in the field of cataract surgery for sometime. The book will also be helpful to optometrists and paramedical people who are concerned with cataract surgery.

Finally, it is my strong opinion that everyone who does cataract surgery should see the case before operation on slit lamp which should be in the operation theater premises for the best performance of surgical steps, and for better visual outcome.

Navneet Toshniwal

Acknowledgments

In the journey of writing this second book, the most important motivation is my first book *Simplified Phacoemulsification*.

Doctors who read this book have appreciated and encouraged me to write another topic relevant to cataract surgery. This force was behind me to present or share some of my practical experience of slit lamp examination and its role in selection and analysis of cataract surgery. These practical experiences, I tried to share in the form of a book, so big thanks to doctors, optometrists, paramedical people who shared their views related to my first book.

From the first day of my practice which I have started in April 1994 and before that, during my undergraduate and postgraduate days, I was observing the work of Dr Sham Toshniwal who is not only my father but also my guide and mentor too. His practical approach towards patients, surgical skills in cataracts was at par. His practical tips helped me a lot to learn and improve my surgical skills. He and his friends Dr Salgarkar Vilas, Dr Jade Arun, and Dr Moholkar Pramod, who have encouraged me to share my views in the form of this book.

It is all time encouragement from my mother, Chand who has motivated me to give knowledge as much as possible and whole heartedly to people. This make me really open up my mind in broad way to share my experience.

My one of the practical teacher Dr TP Lahane, Dean, JJ Group of Hospitals, Mumbai, Maharashtra, India, from whom I have learned academic and nonacademic things concerned with the field of ophthalmology. I am deeply indebted and obliged to Dr TP Lahane for writing foreword for the book.

I am deeply indebted to Dr Neeta, Dr Nilesh, my younger brother Dr Nitin, Dr Kirti, and Dr Murli, who have encouraged and motivated me throughout this journey.

My wife, Sunita was a real backbone and support to me to do this work. My elder uncle Vitthaldasji, Hanumandasji Toshniwal and all Toshniwal family members support was also encouraging me.

In completion of this book Dr Monika Garg who was my Fellow from Rajasthan, had taken a lot of efforts. My friends Dr Dilip Shirsikar, Dr S Jayaram, Dr Mohamed Nassr (UK), Mr Nilesh Pundkar, who is a senior optometrist and my elder son Nikhil who is studying MBBS in Smt. Kashibai Navale Medical College and General Hospital, Maharashtra, India, has also helped a lot for organizing this work.

My special thanks to Mr Ravi and Mr Kunal Mehra from Mehra Eyetech Pvt Ltd, Mumbai, Maharashtra, India, who has provided Topcon slit lamp with built-in camera. All slit lamp photographs were taken from this slit lamp.

I am heartly thankful to Shri Jitendar P Vij (Group Chairman), Mr Ankit Vij (Group President), Tarun Duneja (Director-Publishing), Sunil Kumar Dogra (Production-executive), Neelambar Pant (Production Coordinator), Akhilesh Kumar Dubey, Vinod Kumar Sharma (DTP Operator), Manoj Pahuja (Senior Graphic Designer) and all concerned team members of M/s Jaypee Brothers Medical Publishers (P) Ltd, New Delhi, India, for helping me to make dreams true of mine to reality in the form of book. Thanks to their editorial efforts to improve the book overall.

I would like to thanks Professor Keshav Shinde who was my teacher during college days. It was great impact of his teaching and notes writing style which help me to write this book in this manner. I am most grateful to Dr Madhusudan Albal, Dr Sham Karwa, Dr Ragini Parekh from Mumbai for their valuable guidance. Thanks to all my colleagues from Solapur Ophthalmological Society for their best wishes, and to my friend Sanjay Dargad and all for their encouragement.

Thanks to Santosh Bhagat and all team of Navneet Hospital, Solapur, Maharashtra, India.

Last but not least, I would like my real thank and gratitude toward our all patients, as without them we could not do this noble profession.

Contents

Section 1: Types of Cataract Related to Anatomy

1. **Normal Cataract**   3
   - Normal Cataract   *4*
   - Immature Cataract   *4*
   - Central Dense Cataract   *5*

2. **Anterior Subcapsular Cataract**   6
   - Central Anterior Subcapsular Cataract   *6*
   - ASC Central and Peripheral   *7*
   - Central ASC and Cortical Cataract   *8*
   - Central ASC and Dense Cataract   *9*
   - Central Small ASC with Cortical Cataract   *9*
   - ASC at Multiple Sites   *10*
   - ASC with Immature Cataract   *11*
   - Tiny ASC with Central Dense and Cortical Cataract   *12*

3. **Posterior Subcapsular Cataract**   13
   - Posterior Subcapsular Cataract   *13*
   - Posterior Subcapsular Cataract with Soft Cataract   *14*
   - Immature Cataract with PSC   *15*
   - Dense Cataract with PSC   *16*
   - Diffuse PSC with Very Soft Cataract   *17*

4. **Posterior Polar Cataract**   18
   - Posterior Polar Cataract   *18*
   - Central Dense PPC Surrounded by Thick Plaque   *19*
   - Posterior Polar Cataract with Posterior Subcapsular Cataract and Cortical Cataract   *19*
   - Dense PPC   *20*
   - Posterior Polar Cataract with no Nucleus   *21*
   - Unnoticed PPC   *21*

5. **Soft Cataract**   23
   - Soft Cataract   *23*
   - Soft Cataract with Adequate Size Nucleus   *24*
   - Soft Cataract with Small Size Nucleus   *24*
   - Soft with Diffuse and Cortical Cataract   *25*
   - Diffuse Soft Cataract with Grade 1 Nucleus   *26*
   - Very Soft Cataract with no Nucleus (Clear Nucleus)   *26*
   - Soft Cortical Cataract with no Nucleus   *27*
   - Soft Cataract with ASC and Cortical Cataract   *27*
   - Soft Cataract with PSC and Cortical Cataract   *27*

- Soft with Immature Cataract 28
- Central Nuclear Cataract 28

6. Mature Cataract 30
- Mature Cataract with Adequate Size of Nucleus 31
- Mature Cataract with Liquefied Cortex 32
- Mature with Hard Cataract 33
- Mature with Cortical Cataract 33
- Nearly Mature with Soft Cataract 34
- Mature Cataract with Small Pupil 35
- Mature Cataract with Hazy Cornea 35
- Mature with Very Hard Cataract 36

7. Hard Cataract 38
- Hard Cataract with Adequate Size of Nucleus 39
- Hard Cataract with Dilated Pupil 39
- Hard, Diffuse and Cortical Cataract 40
- Very Hard Cataract 41
- Hard Cataract with PSC 41
- Hard Cataract with Hazy Cornea 42
- Central Hard Cataract 43
- Hard Cataract with Big Size Nucleus 43
- Very Hard Cataract with Brown and Black Color 44
- Very Hard Cataract 45
- Hard Nucleus with Diffuse Cataract 45
- Hard Cataract with Small Pupil 46
- Hard Nucleus with Mature Cataract 47
- Hard Cataract with Shallow Anterior Chamber 48
- Very Hard Cataract 48
- Very Hard Cataract with Calcified Anterior Capsule 49

8. Cataract with Small Size Nucleus 51
- Nuclear Cataract 51
- Immature Cataract 52
- Hard Cataract 53
- Soft Cataract 54

9. Cataract with Big Size Nucleus 55
- Hard Cataract with Semidilated Pupil 55
- Diffuse Cataract 56
- Dense Cataract with Semidilated Pupil 57
- Soft Cataract 58

10. Cataract with no Nucleus 59
- Immature Cataract 59
- Cortical Cataract 60
- ASC with Cortical and Diffuse Cataract 60
- Diffuse Cataract 60
- Posterior Subcapsular Cataract 61

11. Cortical Cataract — 62
- Cortical Cataract 63
- Cortical Cataract with no Nucleus 63
- Cortical Cataract with Grade One Nucleus 63
- Cortical Cataract with Dense Nucleus 64
- Cortical Cataract with Grade 1–2 Nucleus 64

12. Diffuse Cataract — 65
- Diffuse Cataract 65
- Diffuse with Very Soft Nucleus 65
- Diffuse with Demarcated Nucleus 66
- Diffuse with Big Size Nucleus with Respect to Pupil 66
- Diffuse with Dense Nucleus 66
- Diffuse Cataract with Soft and Small Size Nucleus 67

13. Cataract with Weak Zone — 68
- Cataract with Weak Zone Inferiorly 68
- Cataract with Weak Zone on Superior Aspect 69
- Cataract with Weak Zone from 10 to 1 o'clock Position 70
- Cataract with Weak Zone with Central Small Nucleus 71
- Cataract with Weak Zone Nasally or Temporally 71
- Cataract with Multiple Weak Zones 73
- Cataract with Weak Zone in Central Area 74

Section 2: Types of Cataract According to Etiology

14. Developmental Cataract — 77
- Different Variety of Developmental Cataract 77

15. Diabetic Cataract — 80
- Typical Diabetic Cataract 80
- Mature Cataract 81
- Soft Cataract 81
- Cortical and Diffuse Cataract 82
- Very Soft Cataract 83
- Central Anterior Subcapsular Cataract 83
- Cortical Cataract 84
- Different Variety of Cortical Cataract 84
- Cataract with Neovascular Glaucoma 85

16. Steroid-induced Cataract — 86
- Posterior Subcapsular Cataract 86
- Dense Posterior Subcapsular Cataract 87
- Diffuse Cataract 87

17. Traumatic Cataract — 88
- Diffuse Cataract with Posterior Synechiae 88
- Cataract with Central Posterior Synechiae 89
- Anterior Capsular Cataract 90
- Traumatic Cataract with Rupture of Anterior Capsule 90
- Traumatic Cataract with Anterior Capsule Rupture 91

- Traumatic Anterior Subcapsular Cataract   92
- Traumatic Diffuse Anterior Subcapsular Cataract   92
- Adherent Leukoma with Posterior Synechiae   93
- Traumatic Nearly Mature Cataract with Posterior Synechiae   93
- Traumatic Cataract with Iridodialysis   94
- Traumatic Cataract with Localized Iridodialysis   95

18. Cataract with Uveitis   96
- Immature Cataract with Posterior Synechiae   96
- Hard Cataract with Posterior Synechiae   97
- Nearly Mature Cataract with Posterior Synechiae   97
- Posterior Subcapsular Cataract   98
- Diffuse Cataract with Keratic Precipitates   98
- Mature Cataract with Posterior Synechiae   99
- Festooned Shaped Pupil with Immature Cataract   100
- Festooned Shaped Pupil with Mature Cataract   101
- Ectropion Uveae with Hard Cataract   101
- Mature Cataract with Patches of Iris Atrophy and Posterior Synechiae   102

19. Subluxated Cataract   103
- Hypermature Cataract with Inferior Subluxation   103
- Hypermature Cataract with Inferior Subluxation and Calcified Capsular Bag   104
- Hypermature Hard Cataract with Inferior Subluxation   104
- Hypermature Intumescent Cataract   105
- Hypermature Hard Cataract   105
- Hypermature Cataract with Inferior Subluxation   106
- Immature Cataract with Minimal Subluxation   106
- Immature Cataract with Subluxation   107
- Posterior Subcapsular Cataract with Subluxation   107
- Immature Cataract with Superior Subluxation   108
- Subluxated Lens and Cataract with Marfan Syndrome   109
- Microspherophakia   110

Section 3: Cataract with Associated Conditions and Factors

20. Cataract with Pseudoexfoliation   113
- Different Variety of Pseudoexfoliation   114
- Pseudoexfoliation with Adequate Size of Nucleus   114
- Immature Cataract with PXE   115
- Pseudoexfoliation Cataract with Small Pupil   116
- Pseudoexfoliation Cataract with Small Size Nucleus   116
- Pseudoexfoliation with Soft Cataract   117
- Pseudoexfoliation with Hard Cataract   118
- Pseudoexfoliation Cataract with Bulky Nucleus   119
- Pseudoexfoliation with Mature Cataract   119
- Pseudoexfoliation with Cortical Cataract   120
- Pseudoexfoliation with Black Cataract   121
- Pseudoexfoliation with Very Hard Cataract   121

21. Cataract with Shallow Anterior Chamber — 123
- Cataract with Shallow Anterior Chamber *123*
- Dense Nuclear Cataract with Shallow Anterior Chamber *124*
- Dense Nuclear Cataract with Hazy Cornea *125*
- Mature Cataract with Shallow Anterior Chamber *126*
- Pseudoexfoliation Cataract with Shallow Anterior Chamber *126*
- Soft Cataract with Shallow Anterior Chamber *127*
- Postoperative Cases in Shallow Anterior Chamber and the other Eye *128*

22. Cataract with Small Pupil — 129
- Immature Cataract with Small Pupil *129*
- Nearly Mature Cataract with Small Pupil *130*
- Hard Cataract with Small Pupil *131*

23. Cataract with Suspicious Weak Zonules — 132
- Cataract with Wrinkle on Anterior Capsule *132*
- Cataract in Post-trabeculectomized Eye *133*
- Cataract with Weak Zone *133*
- Very Hard Cataract *134*
- Hypermature Cataract with Fibrotic Anterior Capsule *134*
- Cataract with Pseudoexfoliation *135*
- Very Old Age Cataract *135*

24. Cataract with Corneal Opacity and Hazy Cornea — 137
- Dense Cataract with Central Corneal Opacity *137*
- Immature Cataract with Peripheral Corneal Opacities *138*
- Dense Cataract with Hazy Cornea *139*
- Dense cataract with Inferior Corneal Opacity *139*
- Hard Cataract with Corneal Opacity *140*

25. Cataract with Different Shapes of Pupil — 143
- Different Pupil with Nearly Mature Cataract *143*

26. Cataract with Hyperopia — 145
- Immature Cataract *145*

27. Cataract with Myopia — 147
- Immature Cataract in Young Patient *147*

28. Cataract with Embedded Foreign Body in the Lens — 149
- Cataract with Embedded Foreign Body *149*

29. Cataract with Floppy Iris Syndrome — 151
- Hard Cataract with Floppy Iris *151*
- Immature Cataract with Floppy Iris *152*
- Mature Cataract with Floppy Iris *153*
- Cataract and Floppy Iris with Hazy Cornea *153*
- Nearly Mature Cataract with Undilated Pupil *154*

30. Cataract with Glaucoma — 156
- Immature Cataract with Glaucoma *156*
- Immature Cataract and Peripheral Iridotomy with Glaucoma *157*
- Central Dense Cataract with Glaucoma *158*

- Cataract with Pseudoexfoliation and Glaucoma *158*
- Cataract with Narrow Angle Glaucoma *159*
- Cataract with Status Post-glaucoma Surgery *159*

31. Cataract with Iris Coloboma — 161
- Iris Coloboma with Immature *161*
- Iris Coloboma with Dense Cataract *162*
- Iris Coloboma with Soft Cataract *163*

32. Cataract with Micro-ophthalmos — 164
- Mature Cataract with Micro-ophthalmos *164*
- Central Cataract with Micro-ophthalmos *165*

33. Cataract with Vitreous Opacities — 166
- Diffuse Cat with Vitreous Opacities *166*
- Vitreous Opacities with Soft Cataract *167*
- Cataract with Vitreous Opacities *167*

34. Cataract with Pterygium — 169
- Cataract with Pterygium *169*
- Immature Cataract with Pterygium *170*
- Hard Cataract with Early Pterygium *170*
- Hard Nucleus with Advanced Pterygium *171*
- Hard Cataract with Pterygium on Both Sides *172*
- Cataract with Pterygium on Both Sides *173*

35. Cataract with Mooren's Ulcer — 174
- Immature Cataract with Mooren's Ulcer *174*

36. Cataract in Post-radial Keratotomy Case — 176
- Cataract in Post-radial Keratotomy *176*

37. Cataract in Post-penetrating Keratoplasty Case — 178
- Immature Cataract in Post-penetrating Keratoplasty Case *178*

38. Cataract in Post-trabeculectomy Cases — 180
- Dense Cataract with Filtering Bleb *180*
- Dense Cataract with Encroachment of Filtering Bleb on Cornea *181*

39. Cataract in Young Age — 183
- Immature Cataract *183*
- Very Soft Cataract *184*
- Diffuse Cataract *184*
- Central Cataract *185*
- Cortical Cataract *186*
- Immature Cataract *186*
- Central Dense Cataract *187*
- Varieties of Cataract in Young Patient *188*

40. Cataract in Old Age — 189
- Hard Cataract *189*
- Soft Cataract *190*

41. Cataract with Uneven Anterior Chamber   **191**
- Both Eyes Adherent Leukoma *191*
- Adherent Leukoma with Cataract *192*

42. Cataract with Wrinkling of Face   **193**
- Cataract with Wrinkling of Face *193*

Index   *195*

Section 1

Types of Cataract Related to Anatomy

- Normal Cataract
- Anterior Subcapsular Cataract
- Posterior Subcapsular Cataract
- Posterior Polar Cataract
- Soft Cataract
- Mature Cataract
- Hard Cataract
- Cataract with Small Size Nucleus
- Cataract with Big Size Nucleus
- Cataract with no Nucleus
- Cortical Cataract
- Diffuse Cataract
- Cataract with Weak Zone

Chapter 1

Normal Cataract

INTRODUCTION

1. This chapter includes how to see the gross view and slit view of cataract.
2. Gross view will give idea about brightness of cornea, anterior chamber depth, dilatation of pupil and type of cataract.
3. Slit examination will give the exact idea about *anterior chamber depth, type of cataract, layers of lens involved (location of the cataract), density of the opacity and most important is density and size of nucleus.*
   Grading of density of nucleus as follows:
   Grade 1: Yellow
   Grade 2: Dark yellow
   Grade 3: Yellowish brown
   Grade 4: Brown
   Grade 5: Brownish black or black
4. Retroillumination is important in immature cataract specially to see the size and location of lesion like anterior subcapsular cataract (ASC), posterior subcapsular cataract (PSC) and posterior polar cataract (PPC).

Significance of Examination

All these different ways of examination are important not only for diagnosis but also for selection of surgical procedure like Phaco surgery/SICS/ECCE. In Phaco surgery the most important criteria according to author is density and size of nucleus in every case to do the nucleus management perfectly.

Section 1: Types of Cataract Related to Anatomy

NORMAL CATARACT (FIGS 1 TO 3)

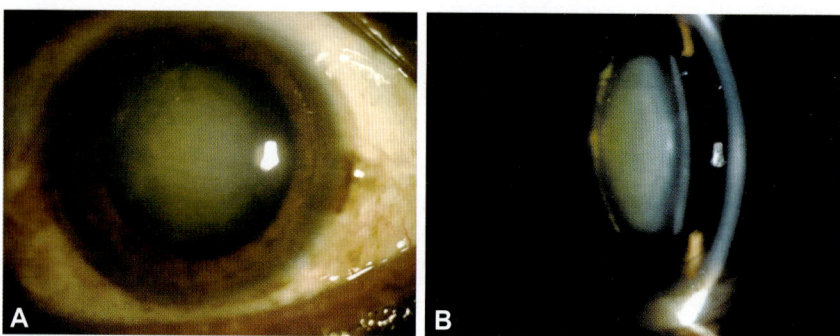

Figs 1A and B (A) Gross view, (B) Slit view

Slit Lamp Examination

Gross View

Central dense cataract.

Slit View

1. All layers of the lens are seen clearly.
2. Grade 2-3 density of endonucleus which is well demarcated and outlined by soft part of nucleus which is grade 2 dense.
3. PSC is also seen.

IMMATURE CATARACT (FIGS 2A AND B)

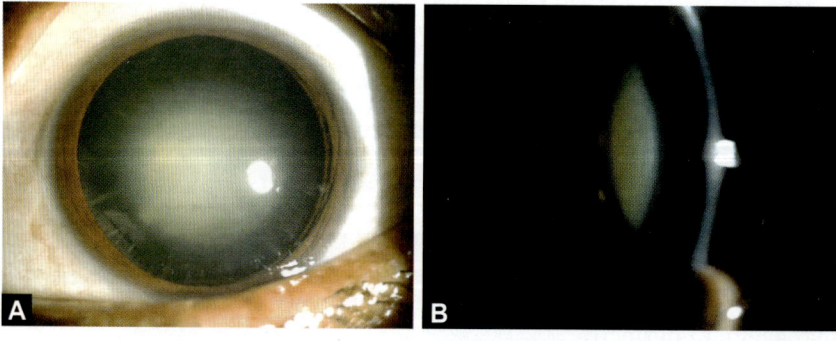

Figs 2A and B (A) Gross view, (B) Slit view

Slit Lamp Examination

Gross View

Immature cataract.

Slit View

1. All layers of the lens are seen.
2. Adequate size of nucleus.
3. Grade 2-3 dense nucleus.

CENTRAL DENSE CATARACT (FIGS 3A AND B)

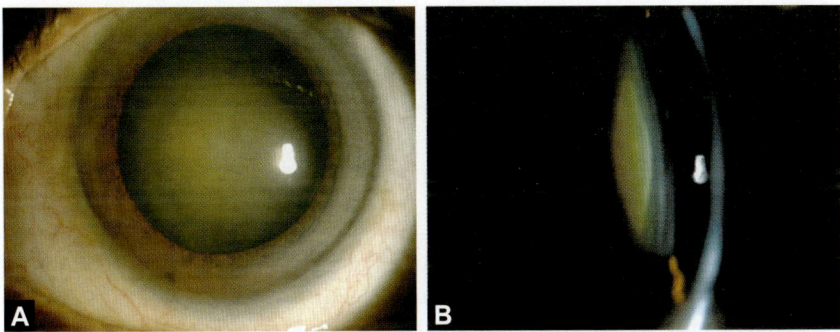

Figs 3A and B (A) Gross view, (B) Slit view

Slit Lamp Examination

Gross View

Central dense cataract.

Slit View

1. All layers of the lens are seen.
2. Thin nucleus.
3. Grade 3 dense nucleus.

Advice

Phaco surgery in such cases is easy and simple (Figs 1 to 3).

KEY NOTE
Normal cataract means the surgeon will feel that it is a straightforward case that can be performed in a simple way with minimal chance of complications.

Chapter 2

Anterior Subcapsular Cataract

INTRODUCTION

1. Anterior subcapsular cataract (ASC) is usually soft cataract situated just beneath the anterior capsule. Common causes are trauma, diabetes, steroid induced and uveitis. This condition is commonly found in young age group.
2. Nucleus management has to be done, as if in soft cataract.
3. Capsulorhexis is most crucial step in these situations which should involve opacified part of the capsule.

CENTRAL ANTERIOR SUBCAPSULAR CATARACT (FIGS 1A TO D)

Slit Lamp Examination

Gross View

1. ASC is in the visual axis.
2. Magnified image reveals details of cataract which is thin at the center and dense at the periphery.
3. This is soft cataract.

Slit View

ASC is confirmed on slit view and retroillumination.

Advice

1. Indication of cataract surgery is not the size of cataract, but it is visual deficit caused by the central location of the cataract in visual axis.
2. Capsulorhexis is most important and difficult step in this case. It can be started at the peripheral part of cataract and this portion of capsule with the underlying cataract should be included in the capsulorhexis.
3. Rest of the cataract management is as in soft cataract.

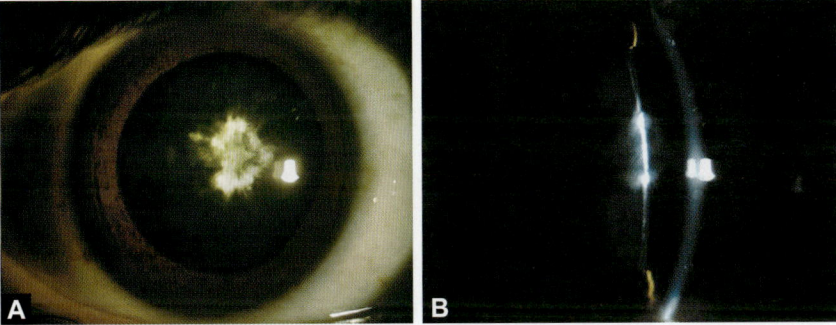

Figs 1A and B (A) Gross view, (B) Slit view

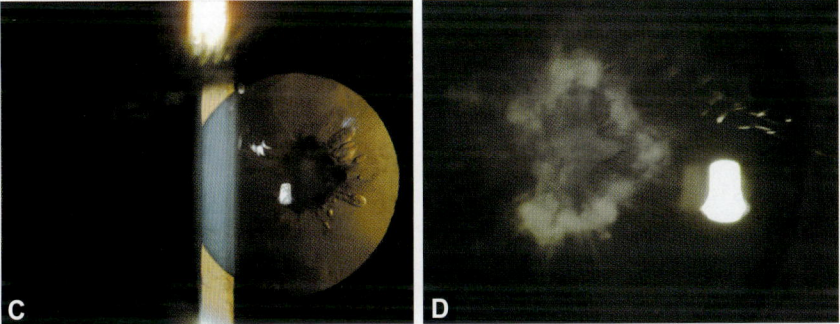

Figs 1C and D (C) Retroillumination, (D) Magnified gross view

ASC CENTRAL AND PERIPHERAL (FIGS 2A AND B)

Slit Lamp Examination

Gross View

1. This ASC is dense in the center and thin at the periphery. Cataractous changes has been pointed towards 8 o' clock and 10 o' clock. This is not localized but it has been spread up to the dilated pupillary margin.
2. This is soft cataract.

Slit View

ASC is confirmed on slit view.

Advice

1. Capsulorhexis is difficult due to peripheral involvement of ASC.
2. Complete peeling of involved anterior capsule is also not very easy but is mandatory.
3. Chances of extension of capsulorhexis are high.
4. Rest of the management is as in soft cataract.

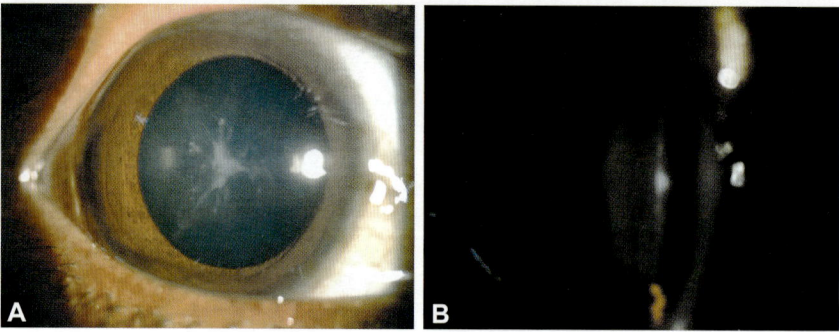

Figs 2A and B (A) Gross view, (B) Slit view

CENTRAL ASC AND CORTICAL CATARACT (FIGS 3A AND B)

Slit Lamp Examination

Gross View

1. ASC is in the center and cortical cataract is in the inferior half of the lens.
2. This is a soft cataract.

Slit View

ASC and cortical cataract is confirmed.

Advice

1. Capsulorhexis with complete peeling of ASC which is relatively easy in this case due to the small area of involvement.
2. Cataract management is as in a soft cataract.
3. Irrigation-aspiration is difficult due to the cortical variety of cataract.

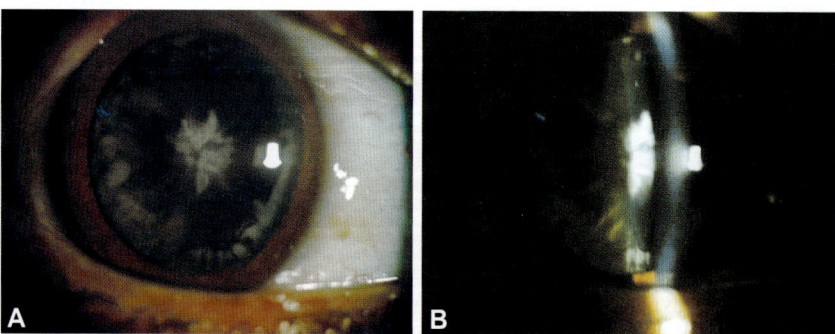

Figs 3A and B (A) Gross view, (B) Slit view

CENTRAL ASC AND DENSE CATARACT (FIGS 4A AND B)

Slit Lamp Examination

Gross View

Grade 2-3 nuclear cataract, cortical cataract and ASC is seen.

Slit View

On slit examination, all these locations of cataract are confirmed and dense PSC is also noted.

Advice

1. Capsulorhexis is crucial due to ASC.
2. Due to grade 2-3 nucleus with adequate size, nucleus management is easy.
3. After the deep trench also, one may not see the red glow due to dense PSC.
4. Division may be difficult due to stickiness of dense PSC.
5. Irrigation-aspiration is difficult due to cortical and sticky cataract.

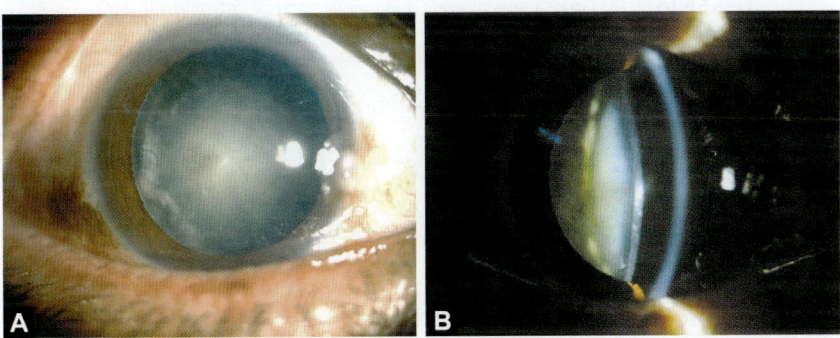

Figs 4A and B (A) Gross view, (B) Slit view

CENTRAL SMALL ASC WITH CORTICAL CATARACT (FIGS 5A TO D)

Slit Lamp Examination

Gross View

Central ASC with cortical cataract.

Slit View

1. Shadow on nucleus is confirmed ASC.
2. Grade 2-3 dense nucleus with adequate size.

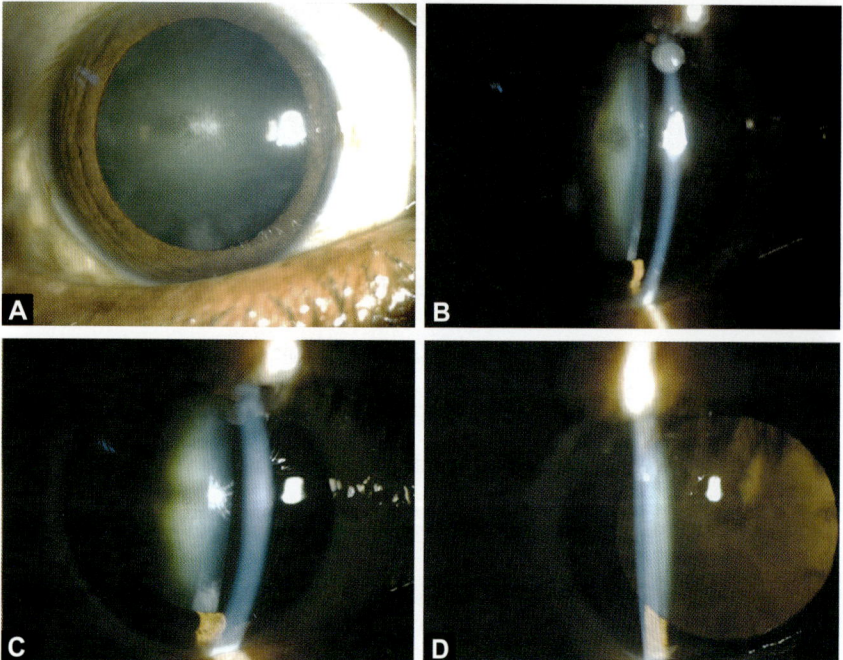

Figs 5A to D (A) Gross view, (B and C) Slit view and (D) Retroillumination

Retroillumination View

Confirmed ASC as a black shadow with PSC and cortical cataract as well.

Advice

1. Capsulorhexis is crucial.
2. Phaco surgery is easy.
3. Irrigation-aspiration may be difficult due to cortical cataract and may take longer than usual time. It means that irrigation-aspiration should be done with patience.

ASC AT MULTIPLE SITES (FIGS 6A AND B)

Slit Lamp Examination

Gross View

ASC in the center as well as at different sites.

Slit View

1. Confirmed ASC at different sites.
2. Shadows on inner structure of capsule of lens confirmed ASC.
3. Soft cataract with big size nucleus.
4. Superior and inferior edges of nucleus are not seen in the pupillary area.

Chapter 2: Anterior Subcapsular Cataract

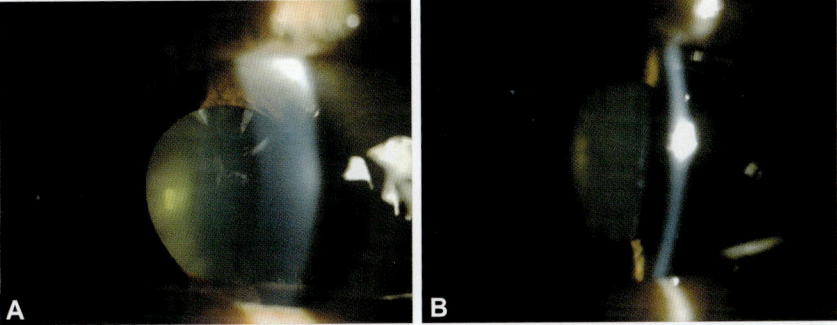

Figs 6A and B (A) Gross view, (B) Slit view

Advice

1. Capsulorhexis is crucial.
2. Phaco surgery is difficult as it is soft cataract and big size nucleus.
3. Modified steps related to soft cataract has to be done in such situations.
4. Irrigation-aspiration is also difficult due to sticky cataract.

ASC WITH IMMATURE CATARACT (FIGS 7A AND B)

Slit Lamp Examination

Gross View

ASC with grade 2-3 nucleus.

Slit View

Confirms ASC with adequate size of nucleus.

Advice

Phaco surgery can be easily performed.

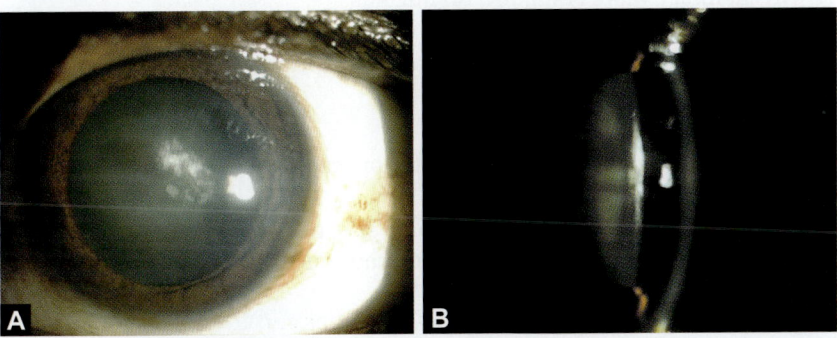

Figs 7A and B (A) Gross view, (B) Slit view

TINY ASC WITH CENTRAL DENSE AND CORTICAL CATARACT (FIGS 8A TO D)

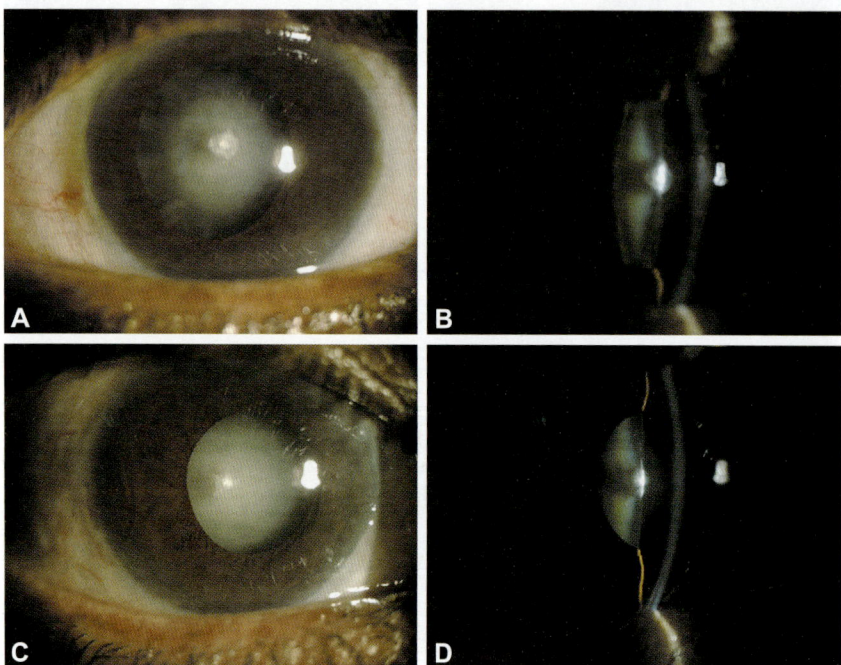

Figs 8A to D (A) Gross view, (B) Slit view of one eye, (C) Gross view of other eye and (D) Slit view of other eye

Slit Lamp Examination

Gross View

Both eyes are showing ASC with grade 3 nuclear cataract with cortical elements.

Slit View

1. On slit image there is shadow on nucleus.
2. Adequate size of nucleus
3. Both ends of nucleus are well demarcated and seen in pupillary area.

Advice

1. In capsulorhexis, peeling of anterior capsule along with lesion is important.
2. Phaco surgery is easy due to adequate size and hardness of nucleus.
3. Irrigation-aspiration should be done cautiously due to cortical variety of cataract.

KEY NOTE

Anterior subcapsular cataract is never a straightforward case as etiology is uncertain, one has to be very careful to tackle this situation.

Chapter 3

Posterior Subcapsular Cataract

INTRODUCTION

1. In this variety cataract involves superficial part of posterior cortex, just beneath the posterior capsule. It may be small or large in size. It may be minimal or dense.
2. This is generally soft variety of cataract. But it can be associated with small nucleus, big nucleus, mature cataract, hard cataract, diabetic cataract, steroid induced cataract, etc.
3. Nucleus management is same as in soft cataract or may be according to associated variety of cataract.
4. Irrigation-aspiration is difficult sometimes due to sticky cataract.
5. Foldable intraocular lens (IOL) as usual.

POSTERIOR SUBCAPSULAR CATARACT (FIGS 1A TO D)

Slit Lamp Examination

Gross View

Posterior subcapsular cataract (PSC) is noticed and confirmed on retroillumination.

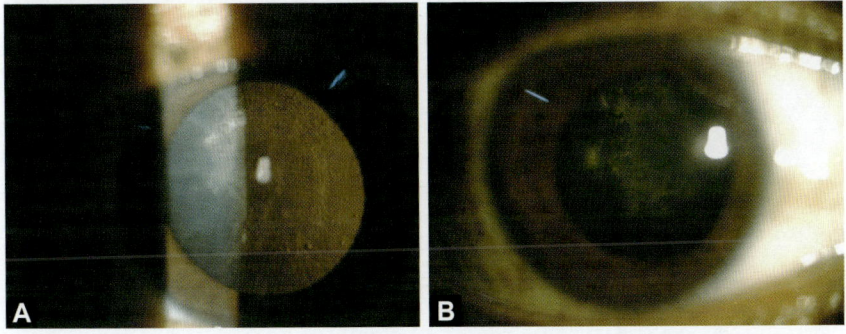

Figs 1A and B

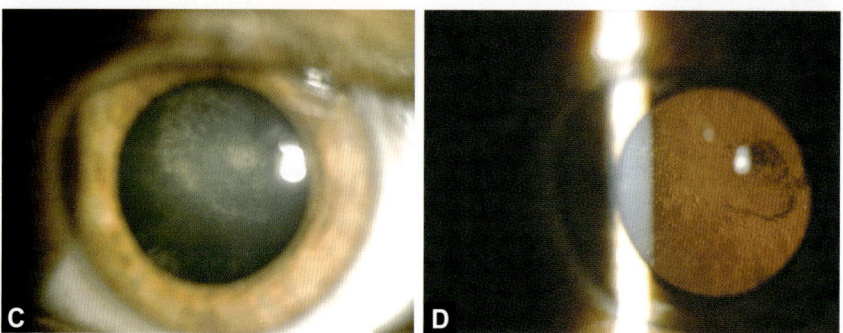

Figs 1C and D
Figs 1A to D (B and C) Gross view, (A and D) Retroillumination view

POSTERIOR SUBCAPSULAR CATARACT WITH SOFT CATARACT (FIGS 2A TO D)

Slit Lamp Examination

Gross View

1. Posterior subcapsular cataract
2. In magnified view, *bread crumb appearance* confirms the posterior subcapsular cataract (PSC).

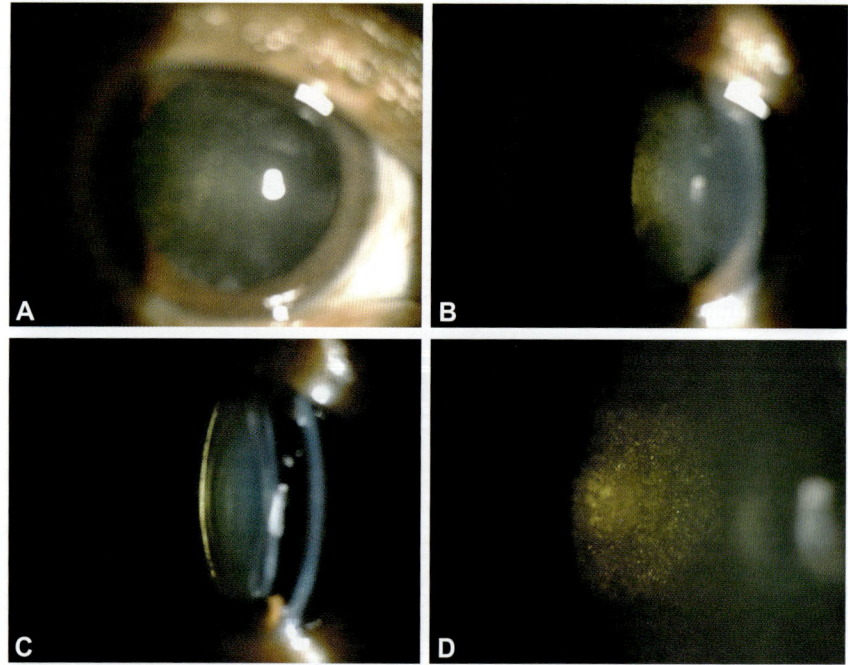

Figs 2A to D (A and B) Gross view, (C) Slit view, (D) Magnified view

Chapter 3: Posterior Subcapsular Cataract

Slit View

1. Layers of the lens are seen clearly.
2. Grade 1 dense and bulky nucleus.
3. Adequate nucleus.
4. PSC is seen as bright illuminated line.

IMMATURE CATARACT WITH PSC (FIG. 3A)

Slit Lamp Examination

Gross View

Immature cataract with PSC.

Slit View

Grade 2 dense nucleus with small size.

Advice

1. After adequate capsulorhexis and hydrodelineation, golden ring will appear around endonucleus part.
2. With viscoexpression this nucleus can be tumbled out of capsulorhexis and can be removed in toto by Phaco surgery.

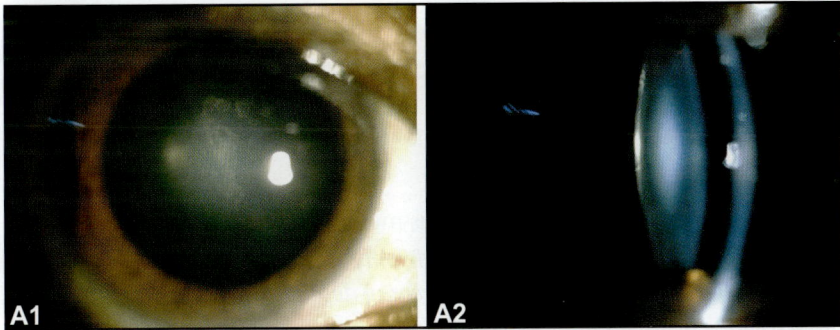

Fig. 3A (A1) Gross view, (A2) Slit view

IMMATURE CATARACT WITH PSC (FIG. 3B)

Slit Lamp Examination

Gross View

Immature cataract with PSC.

Slit View

1. Grade 2 dense bulky nucleus.
2. Adequate size nucleus.
3. PSC is seen as illuminated line at posterior capsule.

Advice

Stop and chop technique is easy to do.

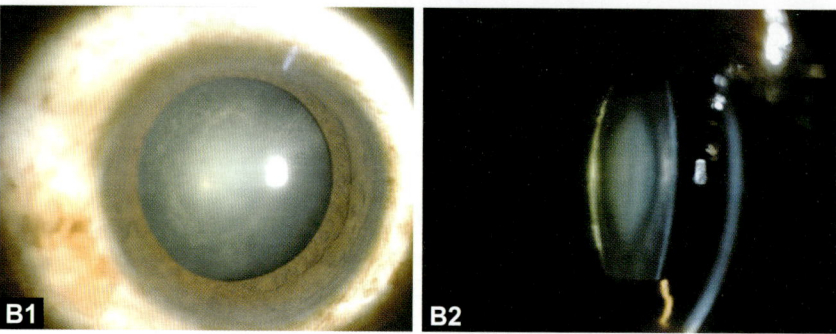

Fig. 3B (B1) Gross view, (B2) Slit view

DENSE CATARACT WITH PSC (FIGS 4A AND B)

Slit Lamp Examination

Gross View

Dense cataract.

Slit View

1. All layers of the lens are seen.
2. Grade 2-3 nucleus.
3. Adequate size nucleus.
4. PSC is very dense.

Advice

1. Stop and chop technique of nucleus management.
2. *Trench: Red glow during the trench may not be seen and should not be considered as end point for assessment of depth due to dense PSC.*
3. Division of nucleus may be difficult due to dense PSC which is usually sticky.
4. Irrigation-aspiration may be difficult due to sticky cataract.
5. Polishing of posterior capsule may be needed in many cases.

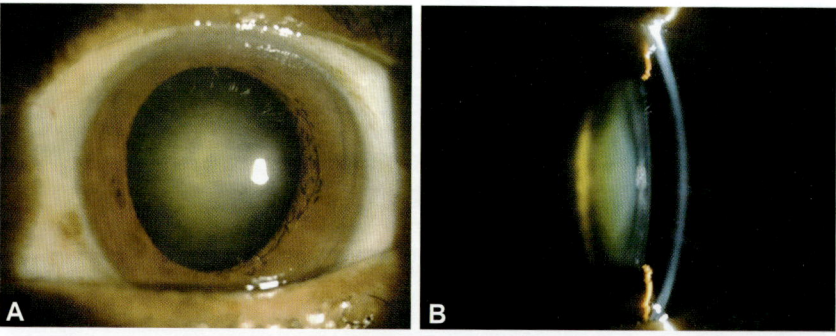

Figs 4A and B (A) Gross view, (B) Slit view

DIFFUSE PSC WITH VERY SOFT CATARACT (FIGS 5A AND B)

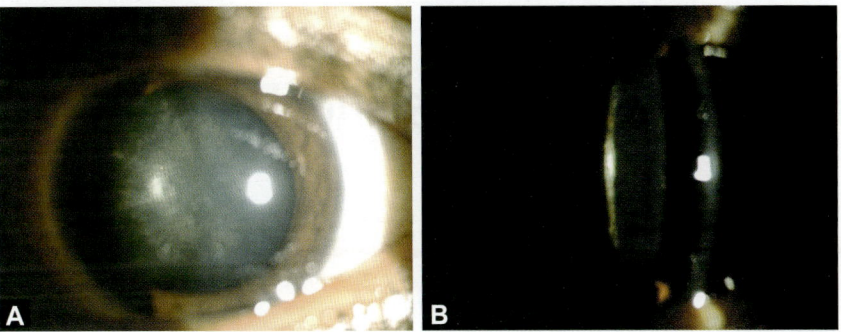

Figs 5A and B (A) Gross view, (B) Slit view

Slit Lamp Examination

Gross View

Posterior subcapsular cataract.

Slit View

1. PSC confirms as bright line.
2. No nucleus.

Advice

In such cases viscoexpression of nucleus can be easily possible.

KEY NOTE
Posterior subcapsular cataract can be associated with weak posterior capsule, whenever surgical steps were performed closer to the posterior capsule, it needs to be very careful movements.

Chapter 4

Posterior Polar Cataract

INTRODUCTION

1. Cataract is situated at posterior pole of the lens. Many times it is attached to posterior capsule.
2. *Many times this plaque like round mass is adhered to posterior capsule. Due to this anatomy, chances of PCR are quite common while doing surgery in such cases.*
3. Usually this is soft variety of cataract where, one can visualize posterior polar cataract easily. *Sometimes this structure is hidden behind mature cataract or hard cataract.*
4. There are many ways to tackle this situation. My way is limbal incision, so that I can convert the case as and when needed.
5. Capsulorhexis should be adequate.
6. Viscodelineation is my choice if cataract is very soft and nucleus is very small. Otherwise stop and chop technique without hydrodissection is important for nucleus management.
7. During irrigation/aspiration, weak central part is to be removed in the end.
8. Foldable intraocular lens (IOL)—one should take precaution of not giving any pressure on posterior capsule during insertion.
9. One should keep ready vitrectomy unit prior to surgery.

POSTERIOR POLAR CATARACT (FIGS 1A AND B)

Slit Lamp Examination

Gross View

1. Posterior polar cataract with layers are seen.
2. Retroillumination is important to confirm and to see exact anatomy of posterior polar cataract (PPC).

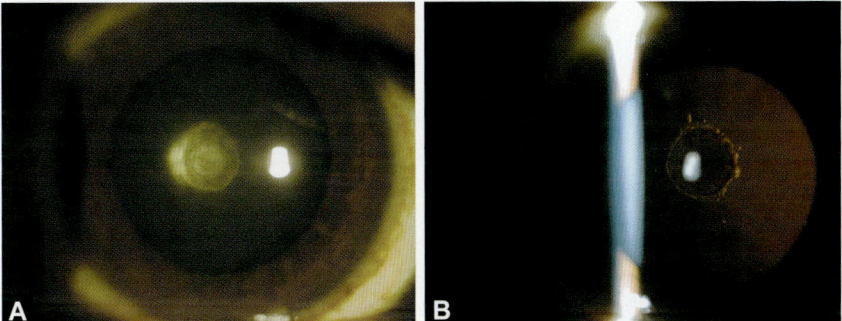

Figs 1A and B (A) Gross view, (B) Retroillumination view

CENTRAL DENSE PPC SURROUNDED BY THICK PLAQUE (FIGS 2A TO C)

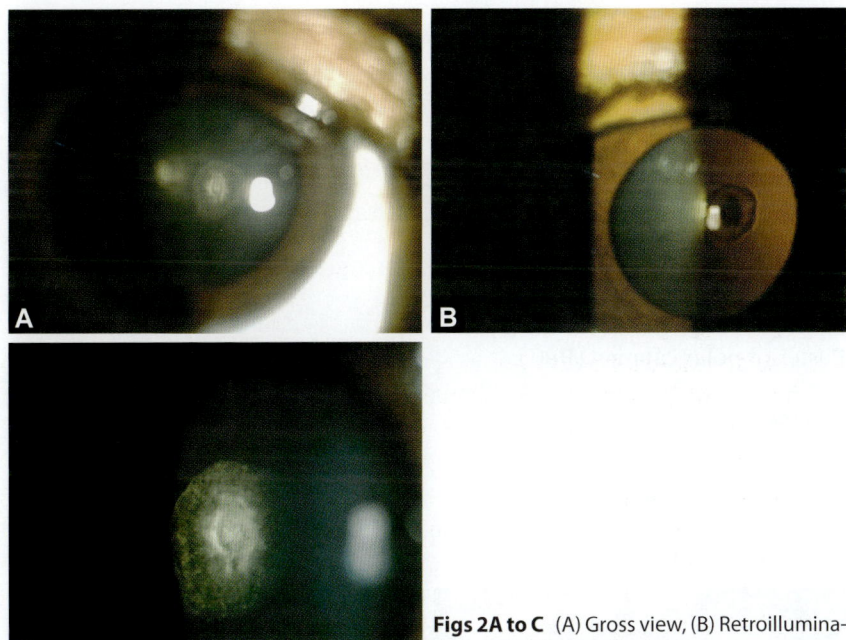

Figs 2A to C (A) Gross view, (B) Retroillumination view, (C) Magnified view

POSTERIOR POLAR CATARACT WITH POSTERIOR SUBCAPSULAR CATARACT AND CORTICAL CATARACT (FIGS 3A AND B)

Slit Lamp Examination

Gross View

Posterior polar cataract (PPC) with posterior subcapsular cataract (PSC) and cortical cataract.

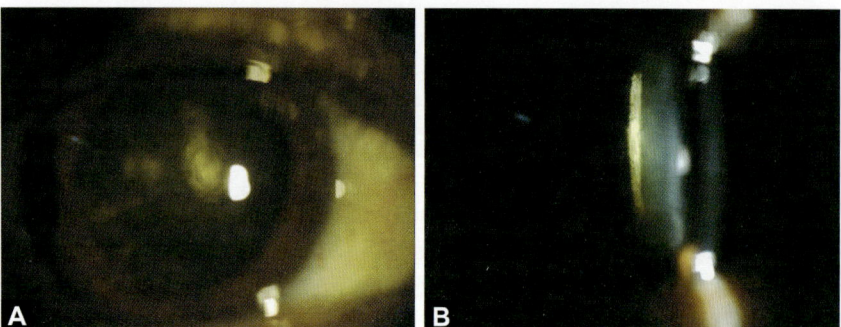

Figs 3A and B (A) Gross view, (B) Slit view

Slit View

1. PPC and PSC confirmed.
2. Grade one nucleus density.

Advice

As PPC is not localized and is associated with PSC, chances of posterior capsule rupture is less.

DENSE PPC (FIGS 4A AND B)

Slit Lamp Examination

Gross View

Posterior polar cataract (PPC).

Slit View

1. Grade 2 dense nucleus.
2. Well demarcated nucleus.
3. Plaque is seen at posterior capsule and adjacent cortex.

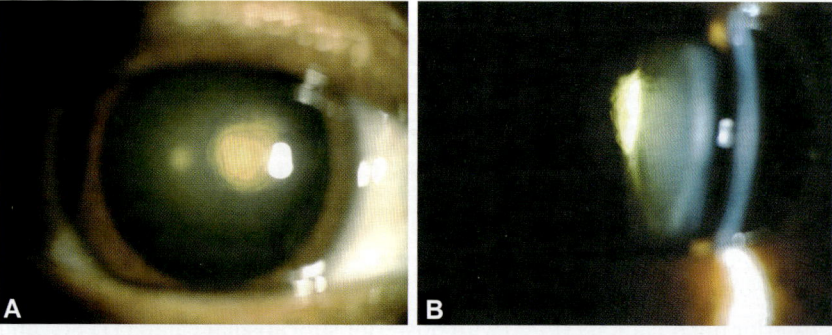

Figs 4A and B (A) Gross view, (B) Slit view

Advice

Stop and chop technique is possible with all precautions of surgical steps needed in PPC.

POSTERIOR POLAR CATARACT WITH NO NUCLEUS (FIGS 5A AND B)

Slit Lamp Examination

Gross View

Posterior polar cataract (PPC).

Slit View

No nucleus.

Advice

Viscoexpression of nucleus is better option.

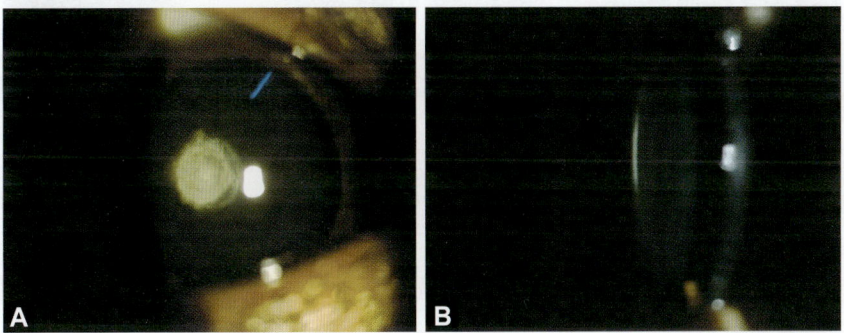

Figs 5A and B (A) Gross view, (B) Slit view

UNNOTICED PPC (FIGS 6A TO D)

Slit Lamp Examination

Gross View

Immature cataract.

Slit View

1. Grade 2 dense nucleus.
2. Adequate size nucleus.
3. Dense PSC

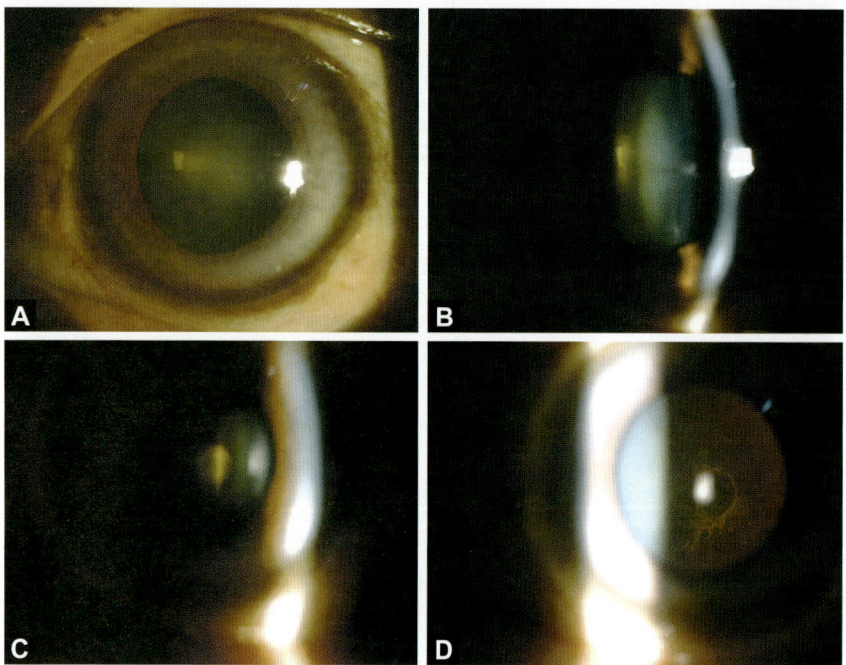

Figs 6A to D (A and B) PPC is not seen, (C and D) In the same case PPC is noticed by changing the direction of slit and confirm on retroillumination

On detailed examination, the surgeon noticed posterior polar cataract which is confirmed on retroillumination.

One can miss this posterior polar component, if surgeon is not in the habit of careful slit lamp examination prior to surgery. This may lead to dificulties during surgery and increases complication rate.

Key Note
Posterior polar cataract is all time challenging situations for every cataract surgeon.

Chapter 5

Soft Cataract

INTRODUCTION

1. This is one of the challenging situations for every Phaco surgeon. Cases seem to be simple but in real way, management differs from case to case.
2. In very soft cataract, viscoexpression of nucleus can be possible.
3. In cases where there is still some mass, routine Phaco surgery procedure can be done.
4. Trench should be small in the center.
5. Division by prechopper as two instruments (sharp instruments) can pass through nucleus substance and may lead to difficulty in division.
6. Hold and lift is very difficult as there is no bulk to hold.
7. Removal of small pieces is easy as there is no big mass to eat and there is relatively more space available.
8. Irrigation-aspiration is always crucial as soft structure is present in the bulk. It takes more time also so patience is needed for this step. Viscoexpression of epinucleus may be frequently required.
9. Intraocular lens implantation is as usual.

SOFT CATARACT (FIGS 1A AND B)

Slit Lamp Examination

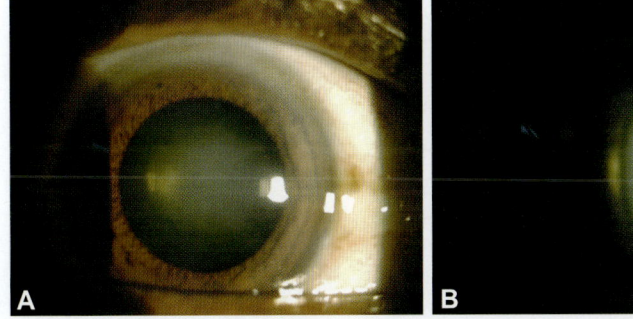

Figs 1A and B (A) Gross view, (B) Slit view

Gross View

Mid-dilated pupil.

Slit View

1. All layers of the lens are seen
2. Adequate size nucleus.

Advice

Routine stop and chop technique can be performed easily.

SOFT CATARACT WITH ADEQUATE SIZE NUCLEUS (FIGS 2A AND B)

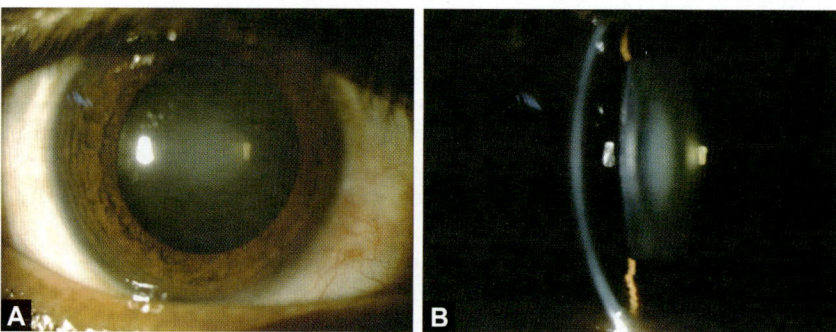

Figs 2A and B (A) Gross view, (B) Slit view

Slit Lamp Examination

Gross View

Soft cataract.

Slit View

1. All layers of the lens are seen.
2. Grade 2 nucleus.
3. Adequate size of nucleus.

Advice

Stop and chop technique is possible.

SOFT CATARACT WITH SMALL SIZE NUCLEUS (FIGS 3A AND B)

Slit Lamp Examination

Gross View

1. Dilated pupil
2. Small size nucleus.

Slit View

Small size of nucleus is confirmed.

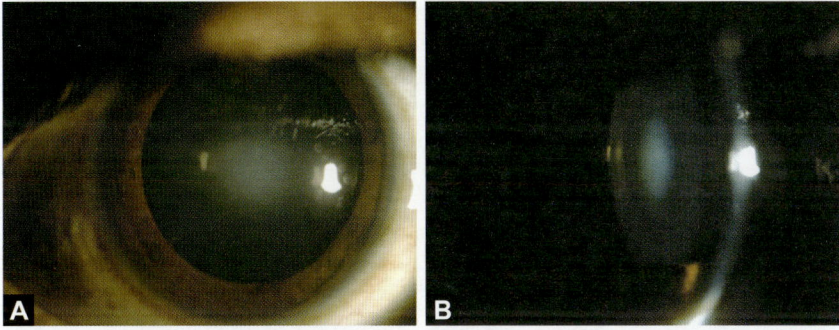

Figs 3A and B (A) Gross view, (B) Slit view

Advice

Big capsulorhexis is possible due to dilated pupil. Viscoexpression of nucleus can be performed.

SOFT WITH DIFFUSE AND CORTICAL CATARACT (FIGS 4A AND B)

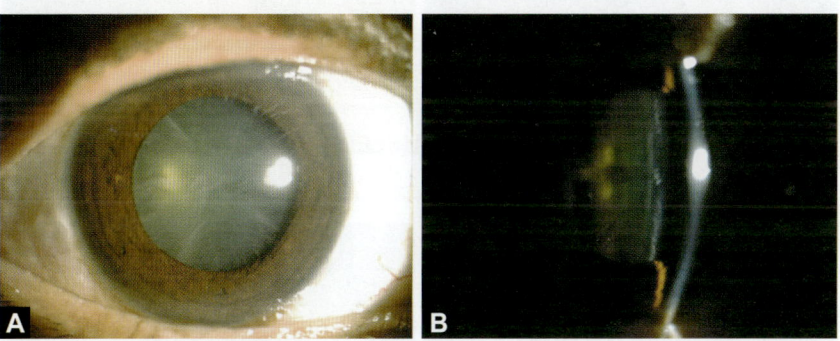

Figs 4A and B (A) Gross view, (B) Slit view

Slit Lamp Examination

Gross View

1. Semidilated pupil
2. Cortical and diffuse variety of cataract.

Slit View

1. Length of the nucleus is big with respect to pupil size.
2. Cortical cataract is confirmed by seeing shadow on nucleus.
3. Element of posterior subcapsular cataract (PSC) is also present.
4. It is grade 1 nucleus.

Advice

1. This condition is usually found in old age, diabetic cases. *This is most crucial condition in soft cataract to tackle.*

2. Stop and chop technique has to be done but would be difficult as the nucleus is very soft.
3. Due to undilated pupil, capsulorhexis is needs to be small.
4. Minimal energy is needed for trench.
5. Division is difficult with Phaco tip and chopper or dialer and chopper, however, division with prechopper is important and easy to do.

DIFFUSE SOFT CATARACT WITH GRADE 1 NUCLEUS (FIGS 5A AND B)

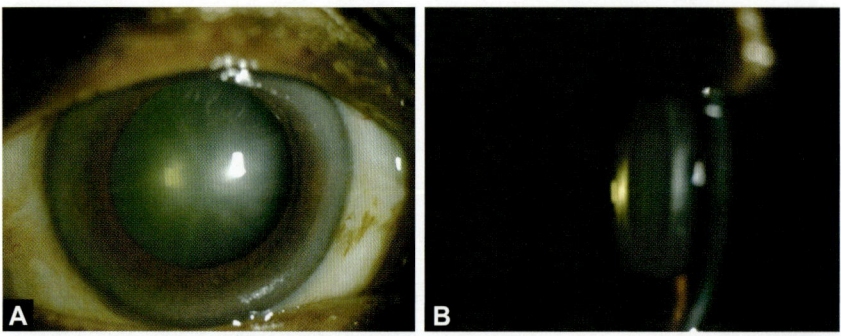

Figs 5A and B (A) Gross view, (B) Slit view

VERY SOFT CATARACT WITH NO NUCLEUS (CLEAR NUCLEUS) (FIGS 6A TO C)

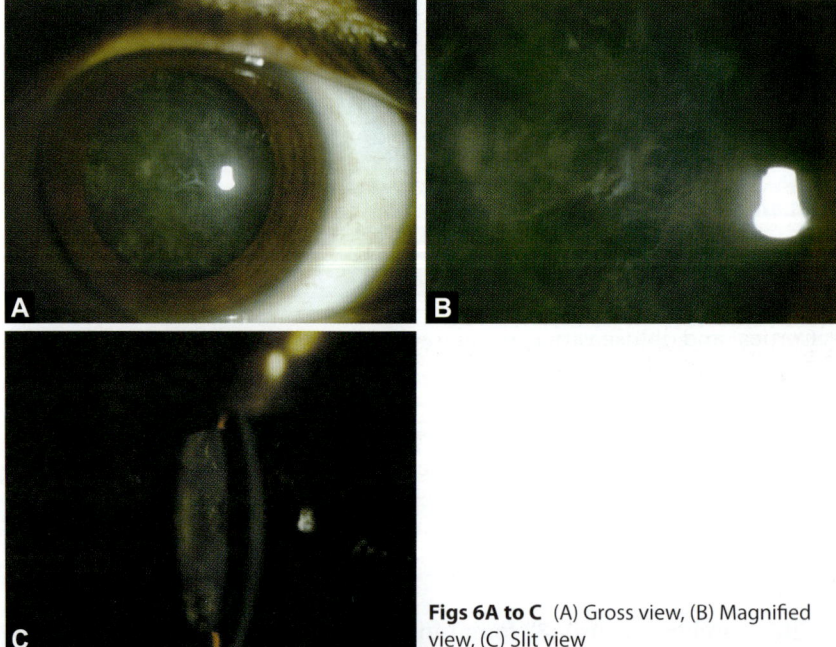

Figs 6A to C (A) Gross view, (B) Magnified view, (C) Slit view

Chapter 5: Soft Cataract

SOFT CORTICAL CATARACT WITH NO NUCLEUS
(FIGS 7A AND B)

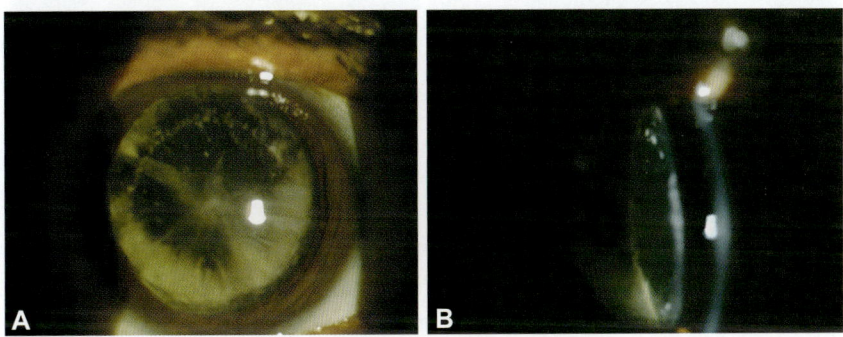

Figs 7A and B (A) Gross view, (B) Slit view

SOFT CATARACT WITH ASC AND CORTICAL CATARACT
(FIGS 8A AND B)

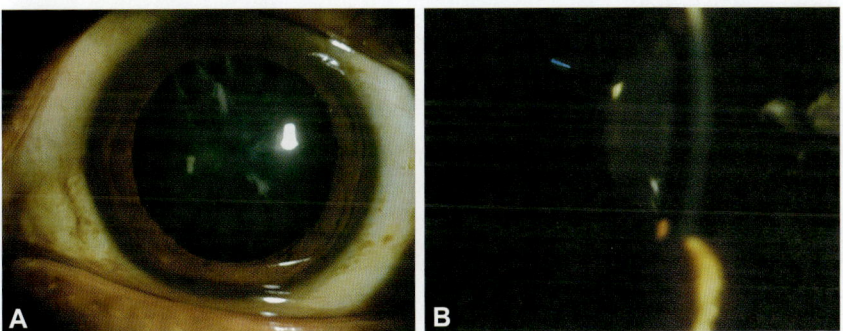

Figs 8A and B (A) Gross view, (B) Slit view

SOFT CATARACT WITH PSC AND CORTICAL CATARACT
(FIGS 9A AND B)

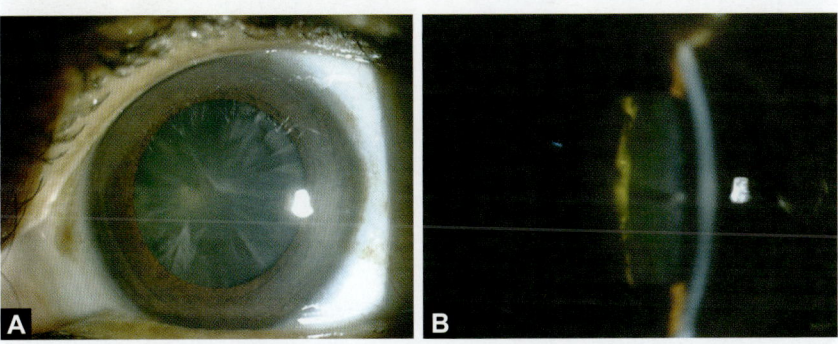

Figs 9A and B (A) Gross view, (B) Slit view

SOFT WITH IMMATURE CATARACT (FIGS 10A AND B)

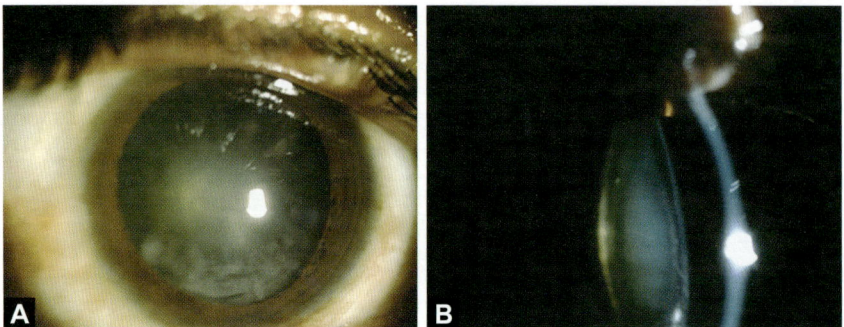

Figs 10A and B (A) Gross view, (B) Slit view

Slit Lamp Examination

Gross View

Immature cataract.

Slit View

1. All layers of the lens are seen.
2. One of the unique thing is that one can see anterior subcapsular cataract (ASC), cortical, nuclear and PSC although it is a soft cataract.

CENTRAL NUCLEAR CATARACT (FIGS 11A AND B)

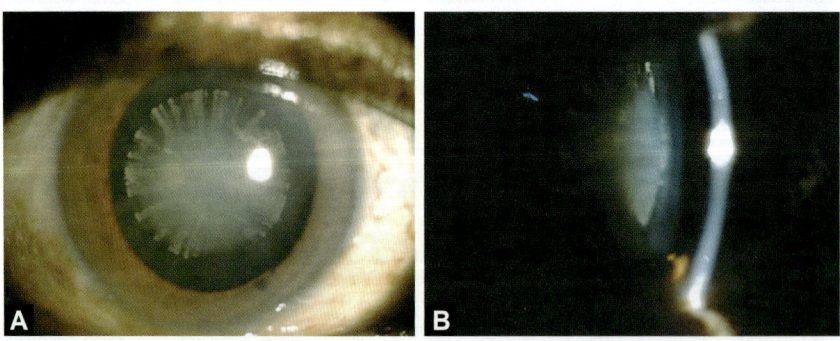

Figs 11A and B (A) Gross view, (B) Slit view

Slit Lamp Examination

Gross View

1. Central cataract
2. Cortical and nuclear cataract

Slit View

1. Grade 1-2 dense nucleus
2. Adequate size of nucleus
3. Cortical cataract is confirmed.

KEY NOTE
Soft cataract is a very common condition in cataract practice which seems to be very easy but in fact it is one of the most challenging situations in Phaco surgery.

Chapter 6

Mature Cataract

INTRODUCTION

1. Mature cataract is a variety of cataract where on gross examination lens seems totally opaque with absence of iris shadow and absence of red glow on examination.
2. It is one of the challenging condition for Phaco surgery and many times conversion to SICS/ECCE is needed.

MATURE CATARACT (FIGS 1A AND B)

Slit Lamp Examination

Gross View

1. Pupil is small.
2. Convex anterior capsule, so capsulorhexis is difficult.
3. Anterior chamber may be shallow.
4. Nucleus may be hard. Nucleus seems to be brown in color.

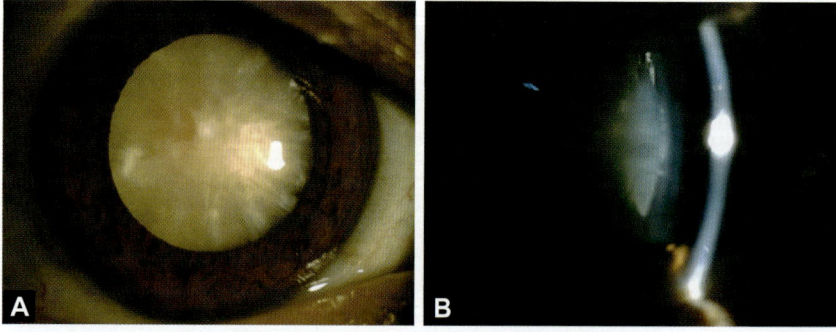

Figs 1A and B (A) Gross view, (B) Slit view

Slit View

1. Slit image define the layers of the lens.
2. Nucleus is hard, grade 4-5.
3. Size of nucleus is very big. Nuclear edges are hidden behind the pupillary area.

Advice

1. As the layers of lens can be seen so phaco surgery can be done.
2. Choice of incision is limbal so that it will be easy to convert to SICS or ECCE procedure if needed.
3. Capsulorhexis should be small. Microcapsulorhexis forceps is better choice to do capsulorhexis. High viscoelastic solutions are preferred.
4. Trench should be in the center. More energy is needed than usual. No hydro procedure before trench.
5. Division may be difficult due to hardness of nucleus. It should be done with the caution as zonules may be weak in this case. Prechopper is important tool for division of nucleus which gives equal pressure on two halves of nucleus.
6. Hold and chop vertical chop or *in situ* chop is important in this situation. Chops may or may not be complete due to hardness of nucleus so partial chops are recommended. Higher parameters are needed for hold and chop.
7. Removal of small pieces more energy than usual is needed. Adequate vacuum in panel or in linear mode and adequate flow rate usually should be In linear mode.
8. Irrigation aspiration should be done with caution as there will be scanty cortex present.
9. Foldable IOL pressure should be avoided in the bag during insertion of intraocular lens (IOL).

MATURE CATARACT WITH ADEQUATE SIZE OF NUCLEUS (FIGS 2A AND B)

Slit Lamp Examination

Gross View

1. Pupil is dilated.
2. Anterior chamber may be normal.

Slit View

1. Layers of the lens are well demarcated.
2. Adequate size and hardness of nucleus is noted.

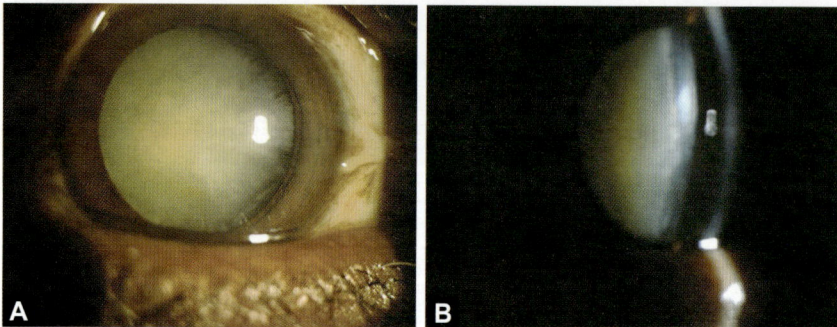

Figs 2A and B (A) Gross view, (B) Slit view

Advice

Routine Phaco surgery procedure with better outcome is expected.

MATURE CATARACT WITH LIQUEFIED CORTEX (FIGS 3A AND B)

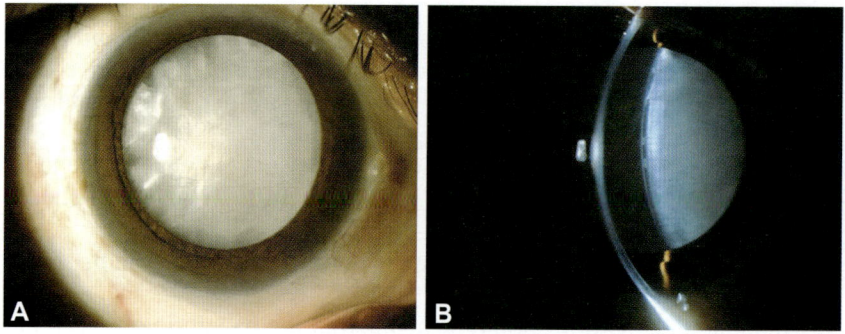

Figs 3A and B (A) Gross view, (B) Slit view

Slit Lamp Examination

Gross View

1. Dilated pupil
2. Liquefied cortex seen.
3. Convex anterior capsule.

Slit View

Layers of the lens cannot be seen clearly behind the anterior capsule.

Advice

1. Phaco surgery is always unpredictable.
2. Capsulorhexis is difficult.
3. Phaco surgery can be possible as nucleus is not very hard.

MATURE WITH HARD CATARACT (FIGS 4A AND B)

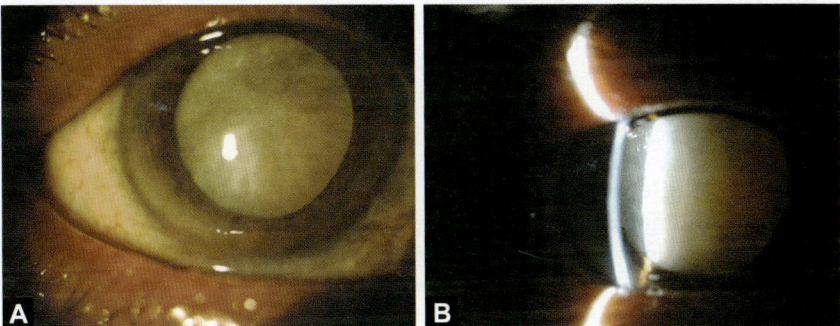

Figs 4A and B (A) Gross view, (B) Slit view

Slit Lamp Examination

Gross View

1. Adequately dilated pupil.
2. Nucleus brown in color. Grade 4 to 5 nucleus.
3. Anterior capsule seems to be weak and thin.

Slit View

1. On slit examination layers of lens are not defined.
2. Size of nucleus is very big as both the edges of nucleus are not visible.
3. Hardness of nucleus is confirmed.

Advice

1. Phaco surgery is very difficult and unpredictable.
2. SICS/ECCE is preferable method.

MATURE WITH CORTICAL CATARACT (FIGS 5A AND B)

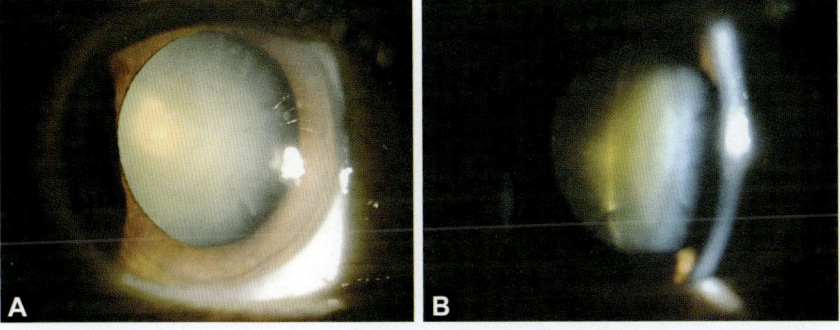

Figs 5A and B (A) Gross view, (B) Slit view

Slit Lamp Examination

Gross View

1. Adequately dilated pupil.
2. Signs of cortical cataract are seen.

Slit View

1. Layers of the lens are well defined.
2. Grade 2 to 3 nucleus which is of adequate size.
3. Edges of nucleus are seen within pupillary area.

Advice

1. Phaco surgery is simple, predictable and easy to do.
2. In irrigation-aspiration some difficulties can occur during cortex removal.

NEARLY MATURE WITH SOFT CATARACT (FIGS 6A AND B)

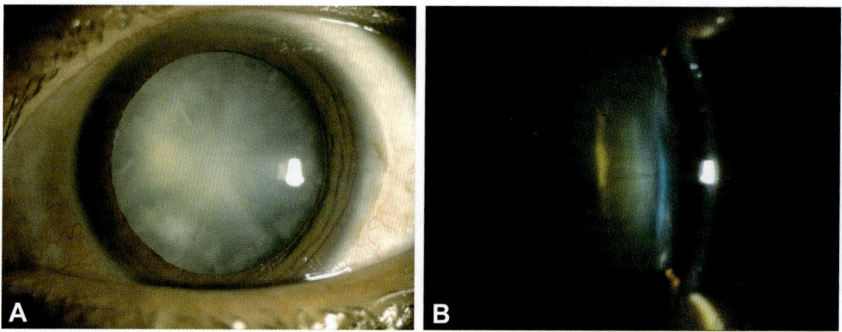

Figs 6A and B (A) Gross view, (B) Slit view

Slit Lamp Examination

Gross View

1. Dilated pupil.
2. Normal AC depth.
3. Cortical cataract.

Slit View

1. Grade 2 nucleus.
2. Size of nucleus is big as compared to the grade of the nucleus.

Advice

1. Capsulorhexis is easy.
2. Phaco surgery is easy.

MATURE CATARACT WITH SMALL PUPIL (FIGS 7A AND B)

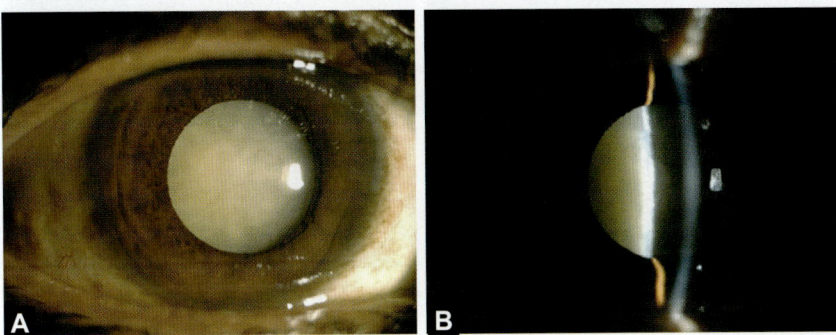

Figs 7A and B (A) Gross view, (B) Slit view

Slit Lamp Examination

Gross View

1. Pupil is small.
2. Anterior capsule is flat.

Slit View

Layers are not seen.

Advice

1. Phaco surgery is unpredictable.
2. Phaco surgery can be possible after following maneuvers
    a. Pupil can be dilated with different techniques.
    b. Capsulorhexis may be difficult.
    c. *First few strokes of trench will give idea about hardness and size of nucleus. Further steps depend on this valuable assessment. This is called as feel of trench.*
    d. *Mature cataract is usually associated with weak zonules so intrabag manipulations should be minimal.*

MATURE CATARACT WITH HAZY CORNEA (FIGS 8A AND B)

Slit Lamp Examination

Gross View

1. Cornea is hazy.
2. Pupil semi dilated.
3. Anterior capsule is fibrotic in the center.
4. May be grade 3 to 4 nuclear sclerosis.

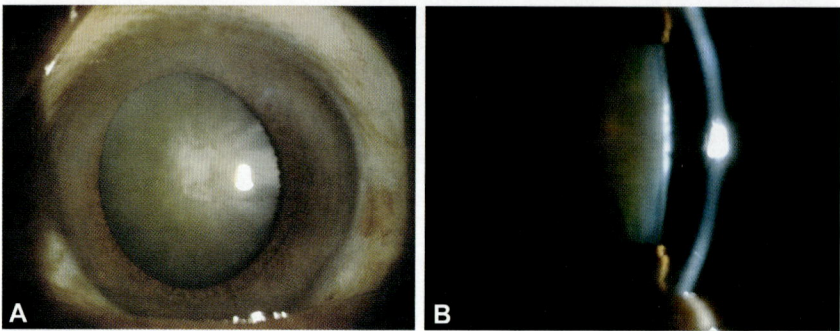

Figs 8A and B (A) Gross view, (B) Slit view

Slit View

1. Layers of the lens can be seen.
2. Hardness of the nucleus is grade 2 to 3 only.
3. Size of the nucleus is big.

Advice

1. Capsulorhexis should be managed carefully due to fibrotic anterior capsule.
2. Phaco surgery is easy to do.

MATURE WITH VERY HARD CATARACT (FIGS 9A AND B)

Slit Lamp Examination

Gross View

1. Dilated pupil.
2. Hard cataract.

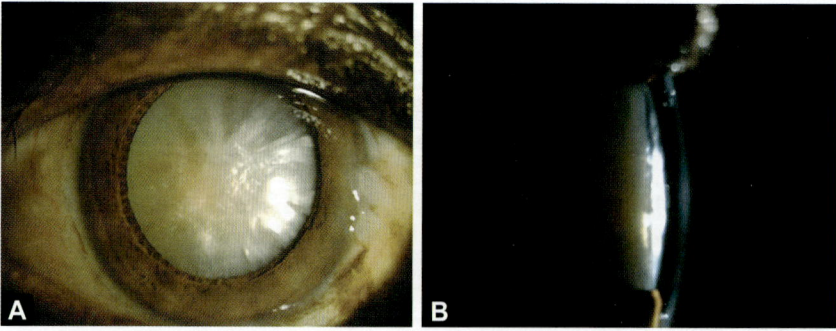

Figs 9A and B (A) Gross view, (B) Slit view

Slit View

1. Grade 3-4. Big size nucleus.
2. All layers of the lens are seen.
3. Convex anterior capsule.

Advice

1. Capsulorhexis is difficult.
2. High molecular weight viscoelastic solution (cohesive and adhesive) can be used throughout the procedure.
3. Wide trench needed anteriorly. Energy should be more than visual. Torsional technology is advised. Both longitudinal and torsional technologies can be used in combination for better cutting. Risk of iris capture is there.
4. Division is difficult.
5. Rests of the steps of nuclear management are as in hard cataract.

KEY NOTE
Mature cataract is always unpredictable cataract surgery by any technique.

Chapter 7

Hard Cataract

INTRODUCTION

1. It is one of the challenging situations in Phaco surgery. Selection of patient for Phaco surgery is important and have significant role for good outcome.
2. *Hard cataract means that grading of nucleus is grade 4 or more. Now selection criteria depend on size of this hard nucleus. Another important factor is its correlation with pupil size. Other factors like corneal haziness, shallow AC are also important for selection of patients and for performing surgery.*
3. Capsulorhexis adequate or big size.
4. Trench is depend upon size and length of nucleus. More energy is needed than usual. Many modifications of design of trench like widening of trench, funnel-shaped trench can be done. Different modes of energy like torsional alone or longitudinal and torsional together can also be helpful. Use of Kelman tip is more important in this situation to avoid vertical gaping of incision during trench.
5. Division most crucial step and one has to learn and master this step.
6. Hold and lift is as usual. Many times vertical chops may be needed in the bag. So combination of vertical and horizontal chops used throughout the procedure.
7. Removal of small pieces step by step removal of pieces is recommended so that space which is formed is really helpful for further maneuvers.
8. Irrigation-aspiration is also crucial as it is degenerated bag. Zonules may be weak.
9. Intraocular lens foldable should be put very gently.
10. *Many times, surgeon may decide to procede with SICS/ECCE or conversion at any stage during Phaco surgery may be required.*

HARD CATARACT WITH ADEQUATE SIZE OF NUCLEUS (FIGS 1A AND B)

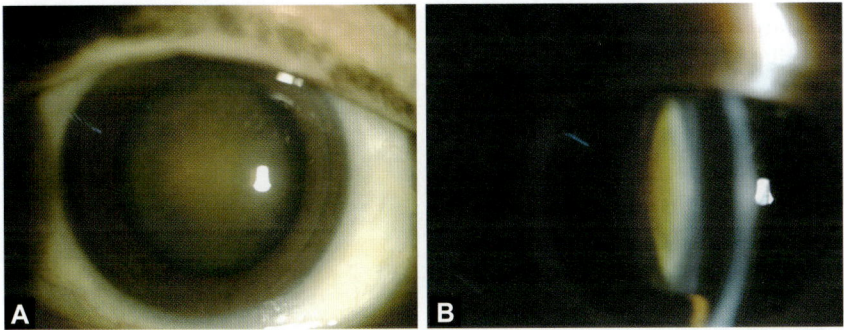

Figs 1A and B (A) Gross view, (B) Slit view

Slit Lamp Examination

Gross View

Hard cataract.

Slit View

1. Dense nucleus confirmed
2. All layers of hard nucleus are demarcated
3. Adequate size of nucleus.

Advice

One can go ahead with Phaco surgery.

HARD CATARACT WITH DILATED PUPIL (FIGS 2A AND B)

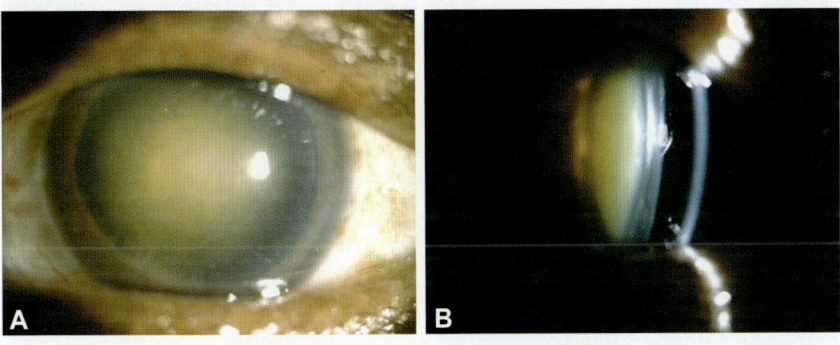

Figs 2A and B (A) Gross view, (B) Slit view

Slit Lamp Examination

Gross View

1. Hard cataract
2. Dilated pupil.

Slit View

1. All layers of the lens are seen clearly
2. Grade 4 dense nucleus
3. Dense PSC is also seen.

Advice

1. Phaco surgery is advisable. Easy to do as all the layers of the lens are distinct
2. Capsulorhexis big capsulorhexis is needed
3. Long trench is needed
4. Division may be difficult as dense PSC is present
5. Hold and lift and removal of small pieces—easy as the layers of lens are distinct which means, there is still space available to perform these steps although it is dense nucleus.

HARD, DIFFUSE AND CORTICAL CATARACT (FIGS 3A AND B)

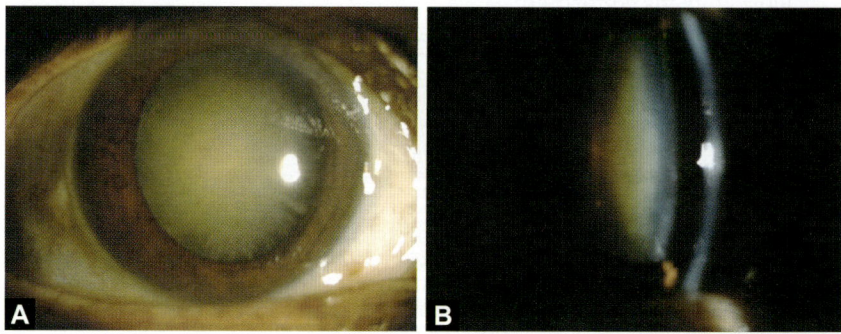

Figs 3A and B (A) Gross view, (B) Slit view

Slit Lamp Examination

Gross View

1. Hard cataract
2. Diffuse cataract and cortical cataract.

Slit View

1. Grade 4 dense nucleus
2. Adequate size of nucleus

Advice

One can go ahead with Phaco surgery.

VERY HARD CATARACT (FIGS 4A AND B)

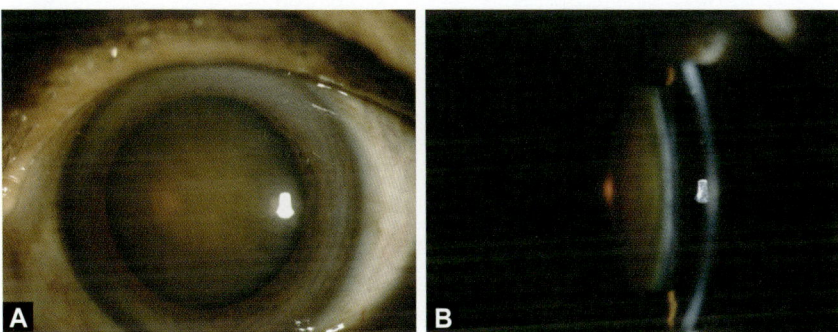

Figs 4A and B (A) Gross view, (B) Slit view

Slit Lamp Examination

Gross View

Very hard cataract.

Slit View

1. All layers of the lens are seen
2. Dense nucleus confirmed
3. Adequate size of nucleus surrounded by sheet of epinucleus.

Advice

One can go ahead with Phaco surgery.

HARD CATARACT WITH PSC (FIGS 5A AND B)

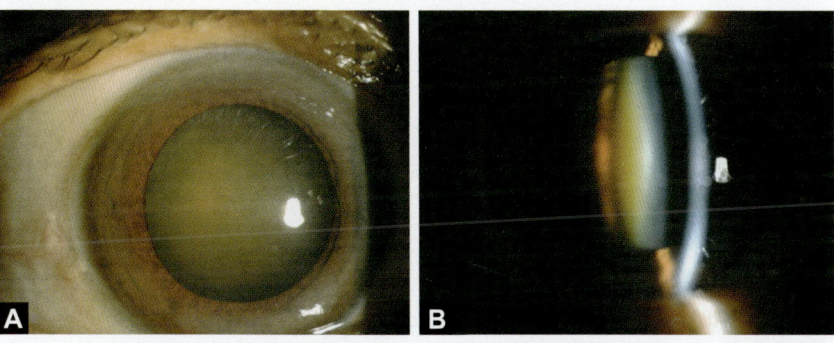

Figs 5A and B: (A) Gross view, (B) Slit view

Slit Lamp Examination

Gross View

Hard cataract.

Slit View

1. Dense nucleus with small size
2. Dense PSC.

Advice

Easy to do Phaco surgery.

HARD CATARACT WITH HAZY CORNEA (FIGS 6A TO D)

Slit Lamp Examination

Gross View

Hard cataract with hazy cornea.

Slit View

Dense nucleus with adequate size surrounded by epinucleus.

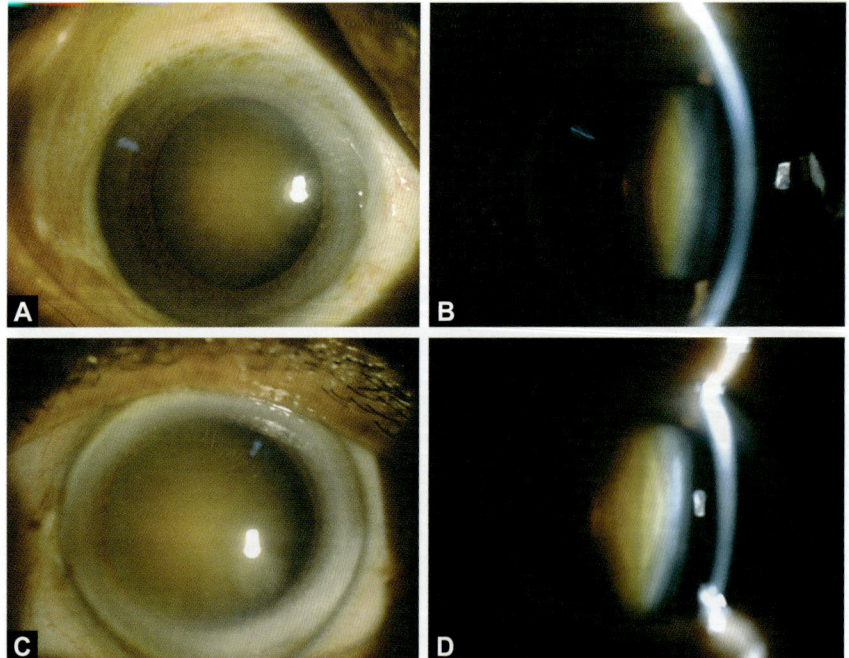

Figs 6A to D (A and C) Gross view, (B and D) Slit view

Advice

One can go ahead with Phaco surgery, if anterior chamber is of normal depth.

CENTRAL HARD CATARACT (FIGS 7A AND B)

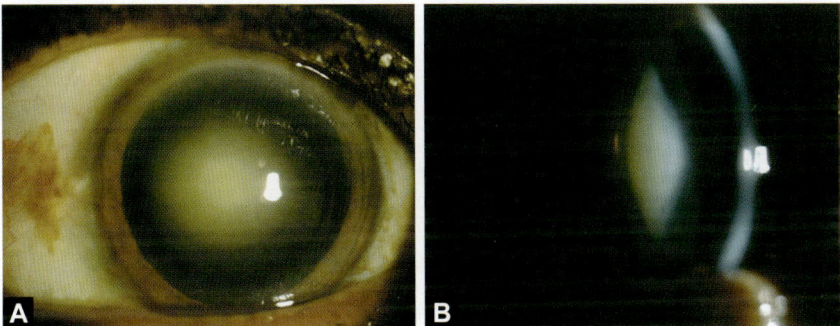

Figs 7A and B (A) Gross view, (B) Slit view

Slit Lamp Examination

Gross View

Central hard cataract.

Slit View

1. Grade 3 dense nucleus
2. Adequate size nucleus.

HARD CATARACT WITH BIG SIZE NUCLEUS (FIGS 8A AND B)

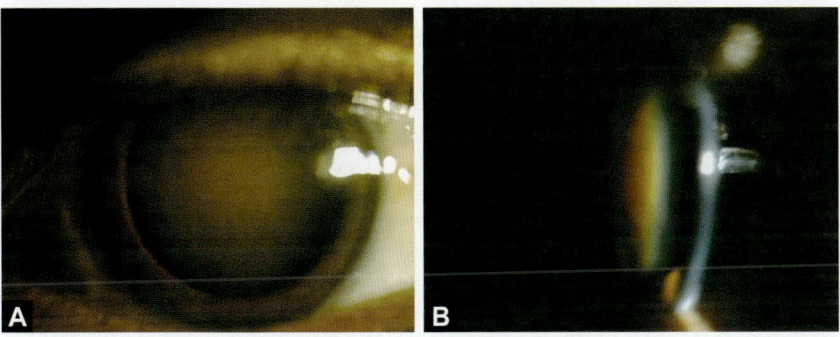

Figs 8A and B (A) Gross view, (B) Slit view

Slit Lamp Examination

Gross View

1. Very hard cataract
2. Dilated pupil.

Slit View

1. Grade 5 dense nucleus
2. Length of nucleus is also long.

Advice

Phaco surgery can be done with caution.

VERY HARD CATARACT WITH BROWN AND BLACK COLOR (FIGS 9A AND B)

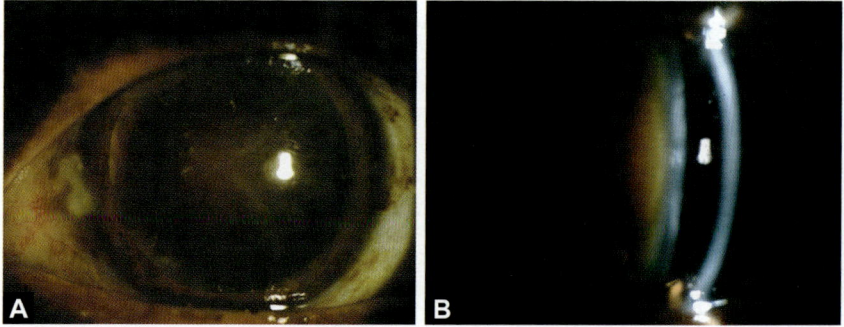

Figs 9A and B (A) Gross view, (B) Slit view

Slit Lamp Examination

Gross View

Very hard cataract.

Slit View

1. Long nucleus demarcated in two parts—central hard core surrounded by semi dense nucleus
2. All layers of the lens are seen.

Advice

One can go ahead with Phaco surgery. *Variable energy is needed according to the density of nucleus.*

VERY HARD CATARACT (FIGS 10A AND B)

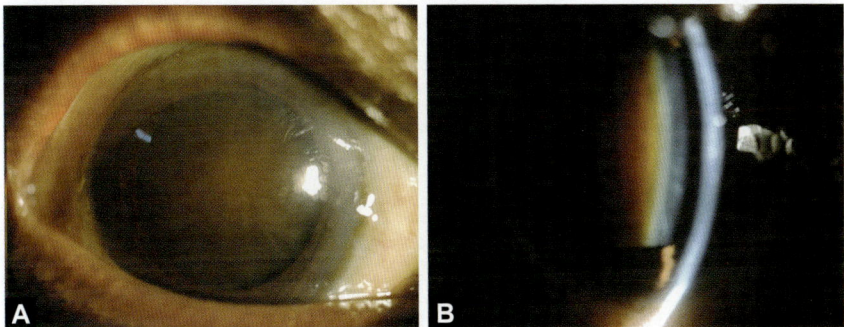

Figs 10A and B (A) Gross view, (B) Slit view

Slit Lamp Examination

Gross View

Very hard cataract.

Slit View

1. Grade 6 dense nucleus
2. Big size nucleus covered by well-demarcated sheet of epinucleus and cortex.

Advice

One can think of Phaco surgery but real expertise is needed.

HARD NUCLEUS WITH DIFFUSE CATARACT (FIGS 11A AND B)

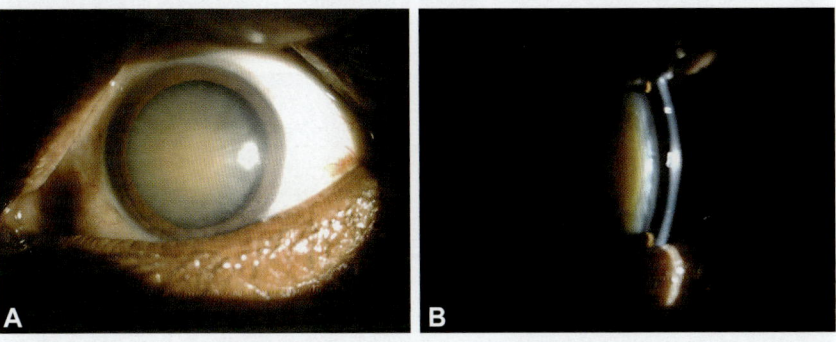

Figs 11A and B (A) Gross view, (B) Slit view

Slit Lamp Examination

Gross View

Hard with diffuse cataract.

Slit View

Dense nucleus with adequate size.

Advice

One can go ahead with Phaco surgery.

HARD CATARACT WITH SMALL PUPIL (FIGS 12A TO H)

Slit Lamp Examination

Gross View

Hard cataract with small pupil.

Slit View

1. Dense, adequate size nucleus
2. All layers of the lens are seen.

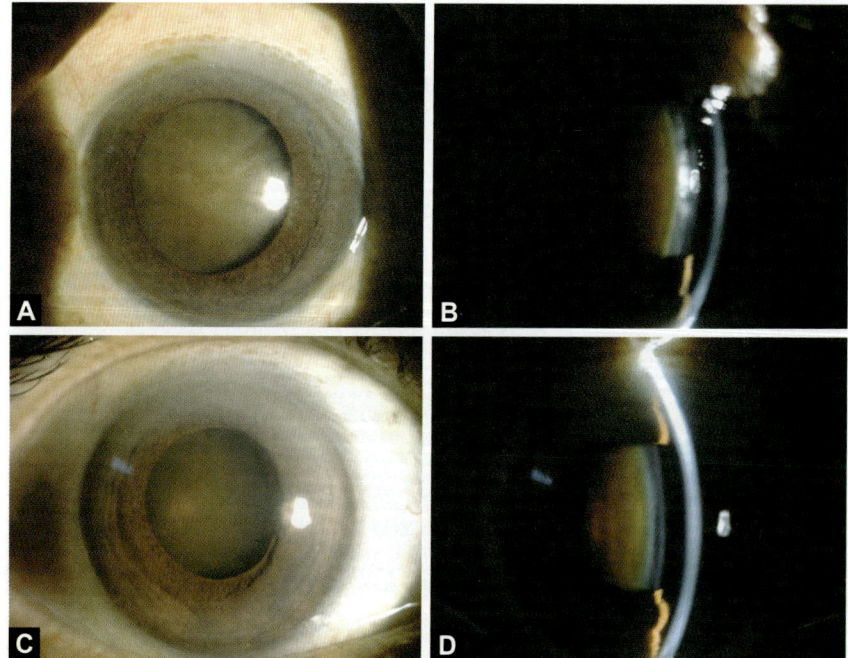

Figs 12A to D (A and C) Gross view, (B and D) Slit view

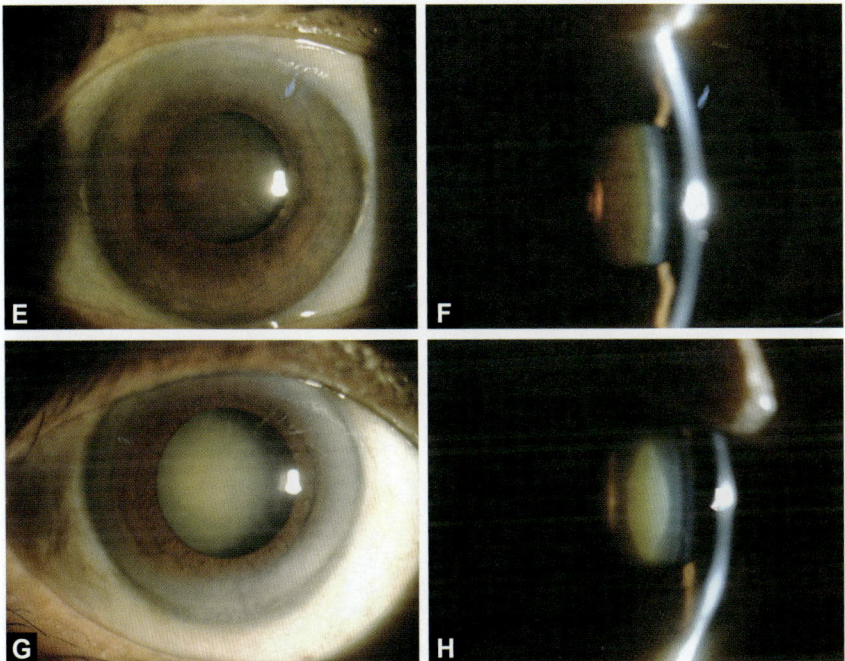

Figs 12E to H (E and G) Gross view, (F and H) Slit view

Advice

With small pupil management, one can go ahead with Phaco surgery.

HARD NUCLEUS WITH MATURE CATARACT (FIGS 13A AND B)

Slit Lamp Examination

Gross View

Hard with mature cataract.

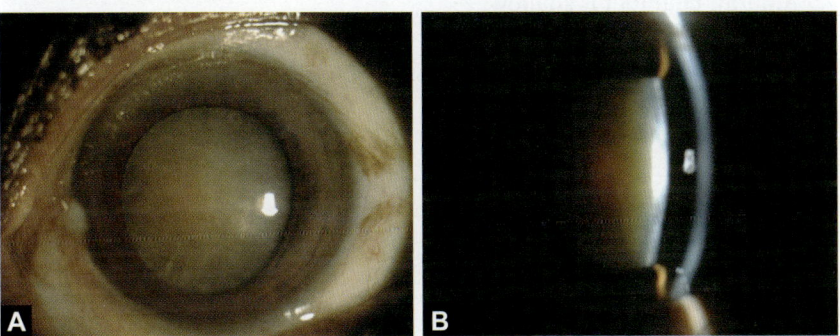

Figs 13A and B (A) Gross view, (B) Slit view

Slit View

1. Big size nucleus
2. Bulky nucleus.

Advice

Phaco surgery is unpredictable but not very difficult.

HARD CATARACT WITH SHALLOW ANTERIOR CHAMBER (FIGS 14A AND B)

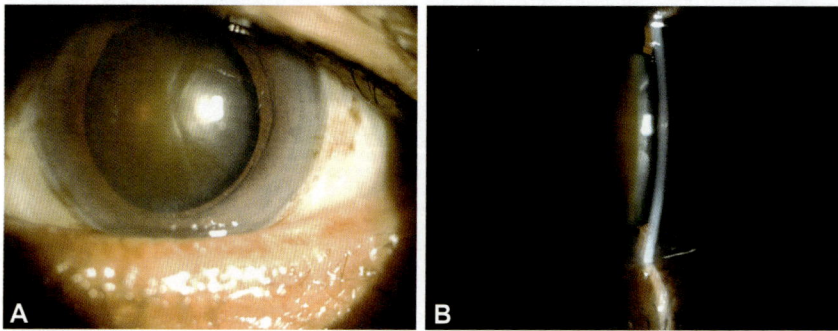

Figs 14A and B (A) Gross view, (B) Slit view

Slit Lamp Examination

Gross View

Hard cataract with shallow AC.

Slit View

1. Dense nucleus
2. Long length nucleus
3. Big size nucleus
4. Anterior chamber is shallow.

Advice

Phaco surgery is possible but due to shallow AC, it is better to avoid Phaco surgery.

VERY HARD CATARACT (FIGS 15A AND B)

Slit Lamp Examination

Gross View

Very dense cataract.

Chapter 7: Hard Cataract

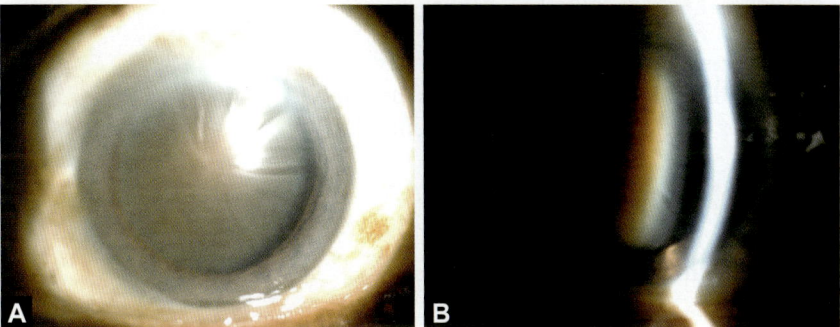

Figs 15A and B (A) Gross view, (B) Slit view

Slit View

1. Grade 6 dense nucleus
2. Bulky and big size nucleus.

Advice

1. Phaco surgery is difficult
2. One can think of SICS/ECCE which is also difficult sometimes.

VERY HARD CATARACT WITH CALCIFIED ANTERIOR CAPSULE (FIGS 16A AND B)

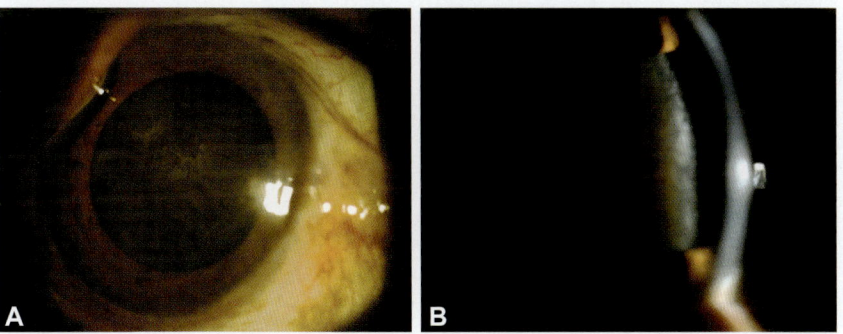

Figs 16A and B (A) Gross view, (B) Slit view

Slit Lamp Examination

Gross View

1. Very hard cataract
2. Calcification of anterior capsule is seen.

Slit View

1. Dense nucleus with grade >6
2. Bulky, big size nucleus, long length nucleus
3. Apex or edges of nucleus are not defined.

Advice

1. One should avoid Phaco surgery
2. One can think of SICS/ECCE.

KEY NOTE
1. *In a hard cataract, one can think of doing Phaco surgery taking in consideration other anatomical factors.*
2. *According to author one has to be very open minded to take decision of conversion to SICS or ECCE at any stage of cataract surgery.*

Chapter 8

Cataract with Small Size Nucleus

INTRODUCTION

1. In Phaco surgery, surgeon is always dealing with nucleus management. It is very practical approach to see not only hardness of nucleus but also size of nucleus. Author is having very strong opinion to consider size of nucleus for better nucleus management.
2. Small nucleus can be soft or hard and may be associated with many other conditions.
3. Surgeon feels more confident to tackle these cataract by seeing slit lamp photographs.

NUCLEAR CATARACT (FIGS 1A AND B)

Slit Lamp Examination

Gross View

1. Grade 2, nuclear cataract
2. Small size nucleus

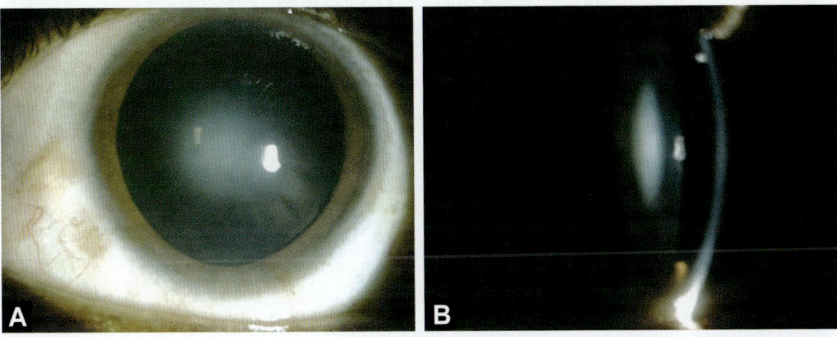

Figs 1A and B (A) Gross view, (B) Slit view

Slit View

1. All layers of the lens are seen
2. Small size of nucleus is confirmed

Advice

1. Phaco surgery is easy
2. Capsulorhexis should be of adequate size 4 to 5 mm
3. Trench should be small in length. Depth of trench should not be too deep. Minimum strokes are needed to complete the trench (if suppose 5 to 6 strokes are needed for every patient, 3 strokes may be enough for this patient)
4. Division should be central and in the mass of nucleus.
5. After lifting of nucleus, no need to chop such a small size nucleus. Direct emulsifying half piece of nucleus in toto.
6. Irrigation-aspiration is difficult because of big mass of epinucleus, so many a times viscoexpression of epinucleus can be done before automated irrigation-aspiration.

IMMATURE CATARACT (FIGS 2A AND B)

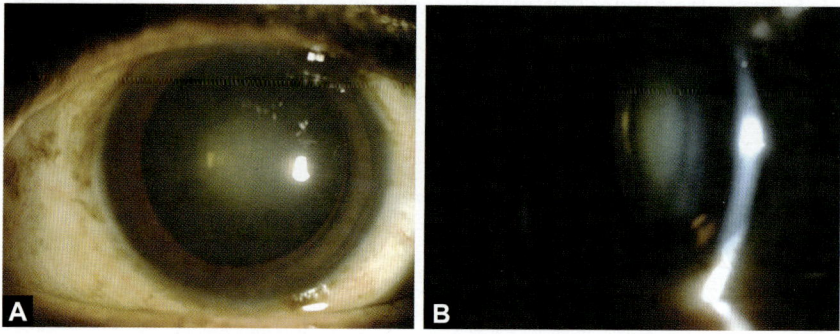

Figs 2A and B (A) Gross view, (B) Slit view

Slit Lamp Examination

Gross View

Small size nucleus.

Slit View

1. Grade 2 nuclear cataract
2. Well-demarcation between nucleus, epinucleus and cortex.

Advice

1. Capsulorhexis should be of adequate size.
2. Hydrodelineation is possible to separate the nucleus from epinucleus.
3. Length of trench should be small. Depth of the trench is half to two-thirds of nucleus. Four-to-five strokes may be needed.
4. Nucleus is more bulky than previous case.
5. Division is easy because of the bulk of nuclear mass.
6. Hold and chop is possible because of mass.
7. Irrigation-aspiration—thick epinucleus has to be removed carefully or viscoexpression of epinucleus may be tried.

HARD CATARACT (FIGS 3A AND B)

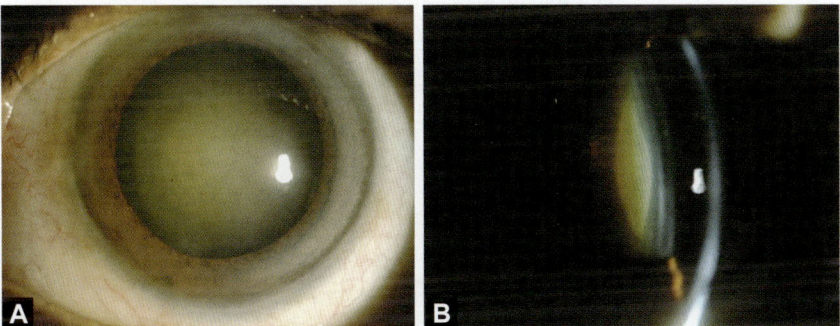

Figs 3A and B (A) Gross view, (B) Slit view

Slit Lamp Examination

Gross View

1. Hard cataract
2. Grade 4 cataract.

Slit View

1. Size of nucleus is small
2. Well-demarcated layers of the lens can be seen.

Advice

1. Capsulorhexis should be 5.0 to 5.5 mm.
2. Trench—although it is a hard cataract, length of the trench should not be more than average. Energy during trench should be more as it is a hard cataract. Trench in this case is safe as nucleus is well surrounded by epinucleus.
3. Division is easy considering the size of nucleus. Sometimes, it may be difficult considering the hardness of nucleus.
4. Hold and chop is easily possible as well as removal of small pieces.
5. Irrigation-aspiration—as usual.

SOFT CATARACT (FIGS 4A AND B)

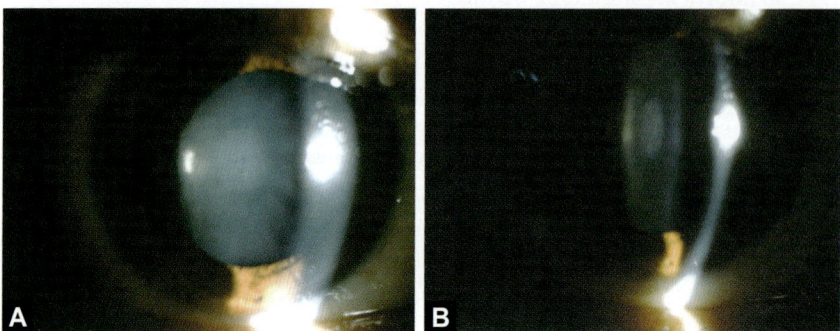

Figs 4A and B (A) Gross view, (B) Slit view

Slit Lamp Examination

Gross View

Very soft cataract.

Slit View

1. Grade 0-1 nucleus
2. All layers of the lens are well-defined
3. PSC is present
4. Some components of cortical cataract is present.

Advice

1. Capsulorhexis should be adequate or big size.
2. No need of Phaco probe as there is no nuclear mass.
3. Hydroprocedure is mandatory.
4. Nucleus can be removed by viscoexpression or by irrigation-aspiration.
5. Irrigation-aspiration of cortex and epinucleus is difficult as it is a big mass due to cortical component.

KEY NOTE
1. Phaco surgery is easy in this situation.
2. Phaco probe movement should be strictly limited to the central zone.

Chapter 9

Cataract with Big Size Nucleus

INTRODUCTION

1. According to the author, consideration of the size of the nucleus is always an important factor for a better outcome in Phaco surgery. It means that small size nucleus is easy to tackle but big size nucleus along with other situation like soft, hard, immature, mature case are always crucial and difficult to tackle.
2. *Generally hard is associated with big size and soft is associated with small size. Sometime there is reverse situation in the cases where soft cataract is associated with big size nucleus which is always difficult to understand and tackle.*
3. Author is considering the big size nucleus in two ways. One is in dilated pupil and when pupil is not fully dilated, i.e. semidiated pupil.

HARD CATARACT WITH SEMIDILATED PUPIL (FIGS 1A AND B)

Slit Lamp Examination

Gross View

Hard cataract with semidilated pupil.

Slit View

1. Grade 4 to 5 dense nucleus
2. Layers of the lens can be seen
3. Edges of the nucleus have gone beyond pupillary area which confirms big size (long length) of nucleus.

Advice

1. Phaco surgery can be performed easily
2. Management of small pupil is needed
3. Capsulorhexis should be adequate or big size
4. Trench should be long in length, and more energy is needed.

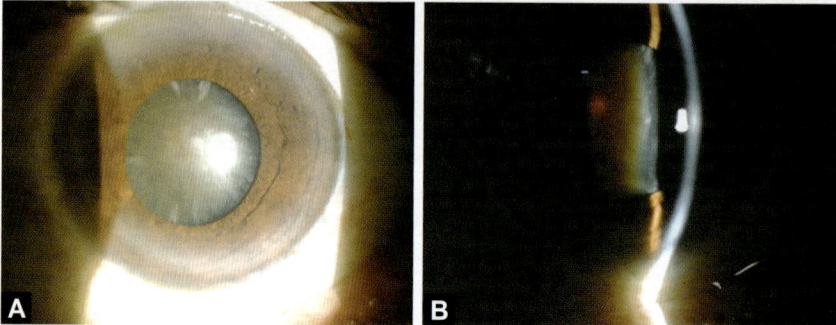

Figs 1A and B (A) Gross view, (B) Slit view

5. Division is difficult to divide, more attempts may be needed
6. Hold and lift and removal of small pieces is as in hard cataract.
7. *Irrigation-aspiration should not be taken lightly as removal of scanty epinucleus or cortex in empty weak bag is difficult.*
8. Foldable intraocular lens (IOL) during insertion, one has to take precaution to avoid pressure on bag.

DIFFUSE CATARACT (FIGS 2A AND B)

Slit Lamp Examination

Gross View

1. Dilated pupil
2. Diffuse cataract.

Slit View

1. All layers of the lens are seen
2. Grade 2 nuclear density
3. Long length of the nucleus.

Advice

1. Adequate size of capsulorhexis
2. Long trench with adequate energy
3. Division is not very difficult
4. *Hold and lift may be difficult during removal of bulky and big half piece of nucleus through the capsulorhexis and also due to soft and sticky cataract.*
5. Removal of small pieces—sometimes energy used is more than needed, which in turn make the cornea hazy
6. Irrigation-aspiration—sometimes difficult due to sticky cataract
7. Foldable IOL implantation—as usual.

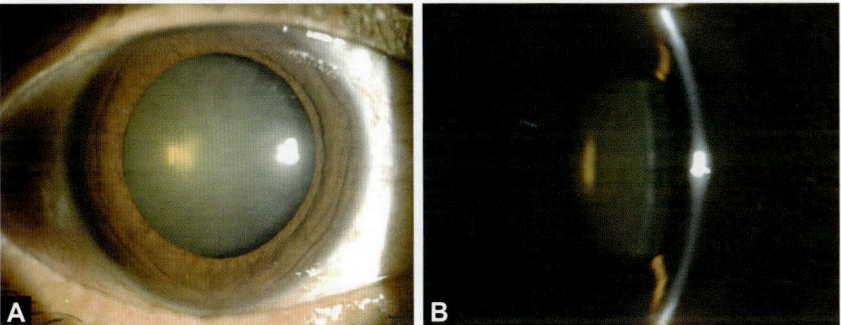

Figs 2A and B (A) Gross view, (B) Slit view

DENSE CATARACT WITH SEMIDILATED PUPIL (FIGS 3A AND B)

Slit Lamp Examination

Gross View

1. Dense cataract
2. Semidilated pupil.

Slit View

1. All layers of the lens are seen
2. Grade 3 dense nucleus
3. Although size of the nucleus is big, central hard endonucleus is very well-demarcated.

Advice

This situation is easily tackled by stop and chop technique.

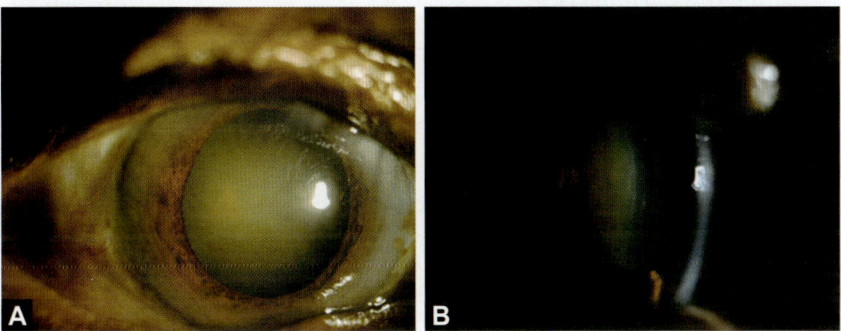

Figs 3A and B (A) Gross view, (B) Slit view

SOFT CATARACT (FIGS 4A AND B)

Slit Lamp Examination

Gross View

1. Mid-dilated pupil
2. Soft cataract
3. *Size of the nucleus seems to be small.*

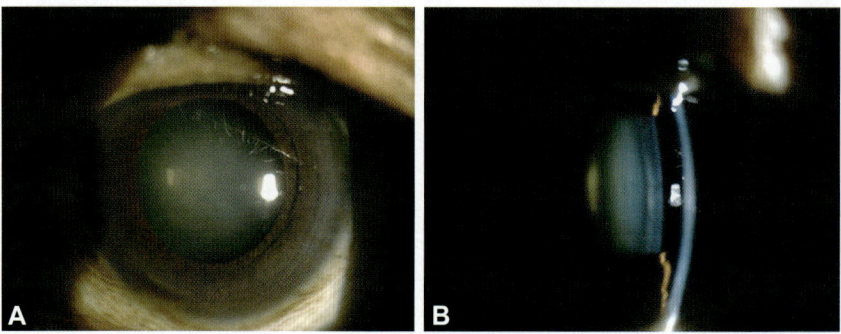

Figs 4A and B (A) Gross view, (B) Slit view

Slit View

1. All layers of the lens are well seen.
2. *Size of the nucleus is big with respect to pupil size.*

Advice

This situation, one has to consider in day-to-day practice as we may not be able to manage the pupil size every time.

KEY NOTE
1. *Cataract with big size nucleus is relative terminology of size of the nucleus with respect to pupil size.*
2. *These cases are not easy to tackle.*

Chapter 10

Cataract with no Nucleus

INTRODUCTION

1. This is unique finding which we have noticed in some of the cataract cases like immature cataract, anterior subcapsular cataract (ASC), cortical cataract, diffuse cataract, posterior subcapsular cataract (PSC), etc.
2. Cataract management is like in soft cataract cases. Use of Phaco tip can be avoided as there is no nucleus.

IMMATURE CATARACT (FIGS 1A AND B)

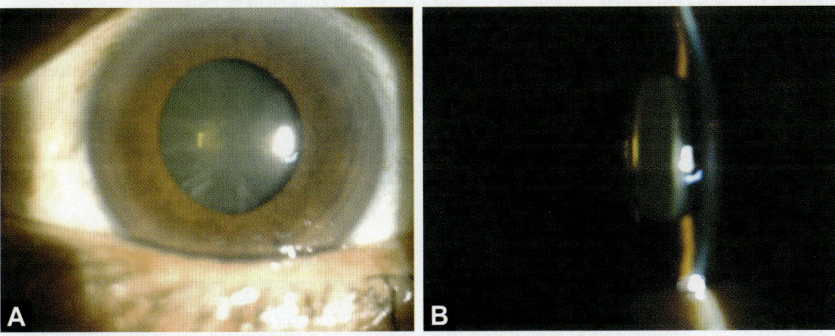

Figs 1A and B (A) Gross view, (B) Slit view

CORTICAL CATARACT (FIGS 2A AND B)

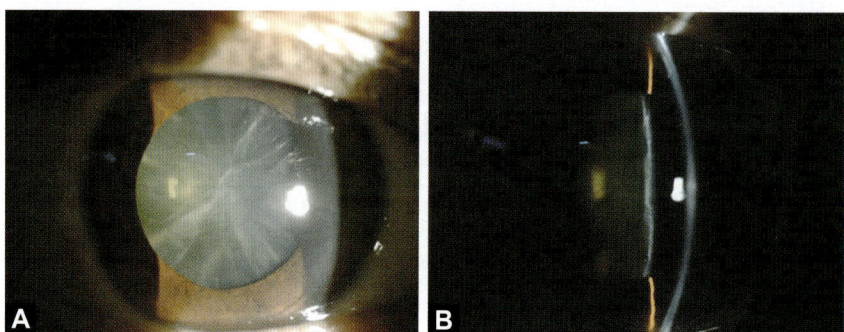

Figs 2A and B (A) Gross view, (B) Slit view

ASC WITH CORTICAL AND DIFFUSE CATARACT (FIGS 3A AND B)

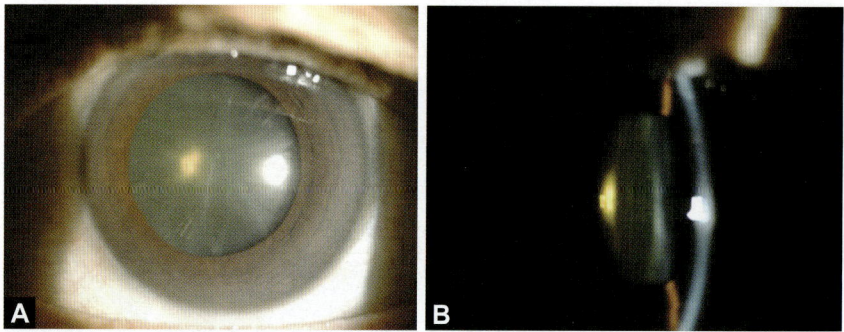

Figs 3A and B (A) Gross view, (B) Slit view

DIFFUSE CATARACT (FIGS 4A AND B)

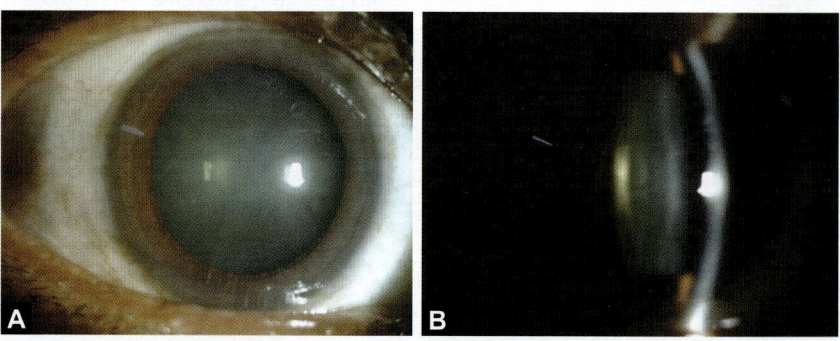

Figs 4A and B (A) Gross view, (B) Slit view

Chapter 10: Cataract with no Nucleus

POSTERIOR SUBCAPSULAR CATARACT (FIGS 5A TO F)

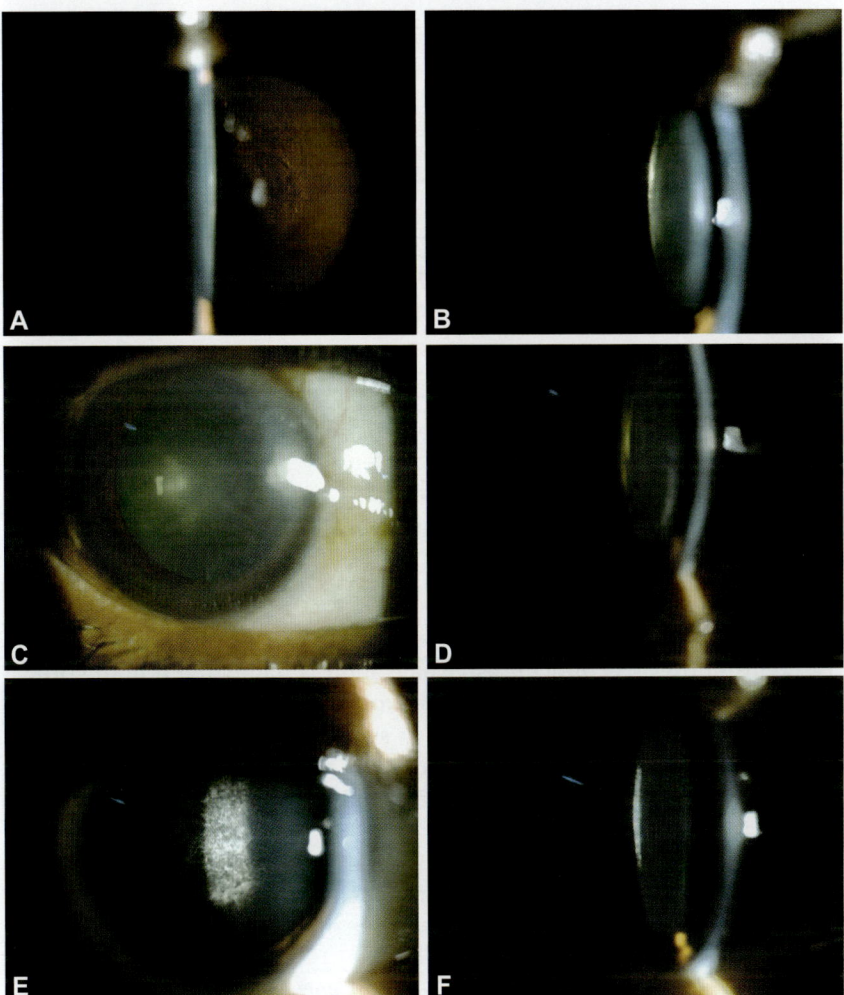

Figs 5A to F (A, C, E) Gross view, (B, D, F) Slit view

KEY NOTE
Cataract with no nucleus means central nuclear area is clear.

Chapter 11

Cortical Cataract

INTRODUCTION

1. Cataract is in the cortical layer of the lens.
2. It is usually soft variety of cataract.
3. Many times diabetes is associated factor.

Steps of Surgery

1. Incision can be limbal or clear corneal.
2. Capsulorhexis is difficult as visualization is hampered due to cortical cataract. Trypan blue dye is needed for capsulorhexis.
3. Hydroprocedures are important in such variety of cataracts for better cleavage and separation of lens layers.
4. Length and depth of trench depend on the size and density of nucleus.
5. Division as a routine.
6. Hold and chop is difficult step in this variety of cataract. These cases are usually sticky cataract. Separation of nucleus with epinucleus is difficult. Chopping may be difficult due to non visualization of the cleavage.
7. Removal of small pieces as usual.
8. *Irrigation-aspiration of epinucleus and cortex is difficult due to thick epinucleus and cortex, sticky tissue, adherence of cortex to capsule and difficult visualization.* Coaxial irrigation-aspiration is superior to bimanual due to large bore size of aspiration port. Subincisional cortex may need bimanual irrigation-aspiration. Chances of blockage of aspiration cannula is quite common. Chopper may be helpful to crush the soft tissue at the aspiration port, which will assist the aspiration. It may take more time, so patience is needed.
9. Complications during irrigation-aspiration—chances of zonular dialysis is there.
10. Implantation of IOL as routine.

CORTICAL CATARACT (FIGS 1A AND B)

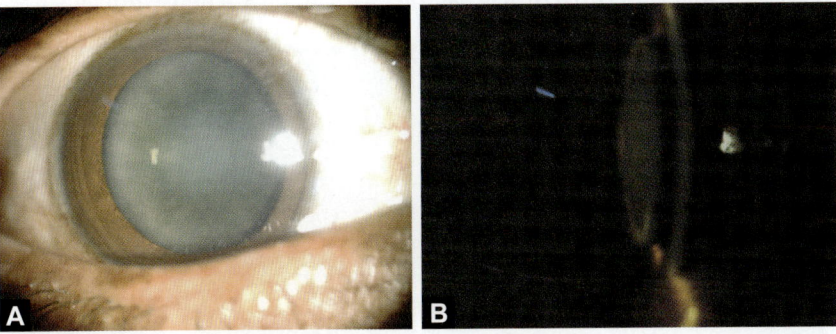

Figs 1A and B (A) Gross view, (B) Slit view

CORTICAL CATARACT WITH NO NUCLEUS (FIGS 2A AND B)

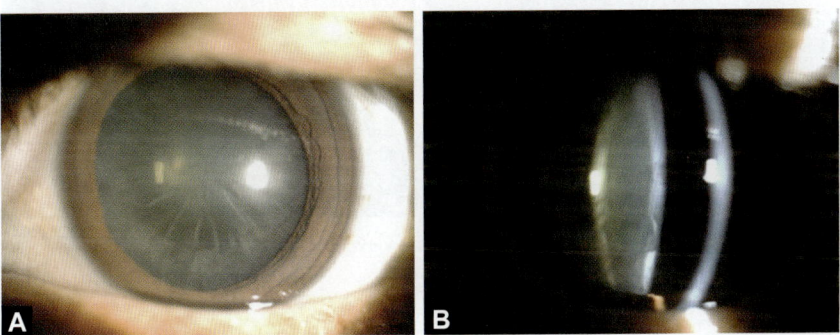

Figs 2A and B (A) Gross view, (B) Slit view

CORTICAL CATARACT WITH GRADE ONE NUCLEUS (FIGS 3A AND B)

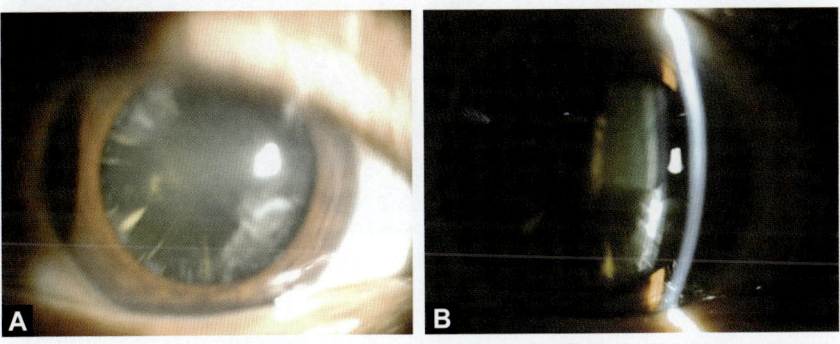

Figs 3A and B (A) Gross view, (B) Slit view

CORTICAL CATARACT WITH DENSE NUCLEUS (FIGS 4A TO D)

This is unusual variety of cortical cataract with grade 3–4 dense nucleus.

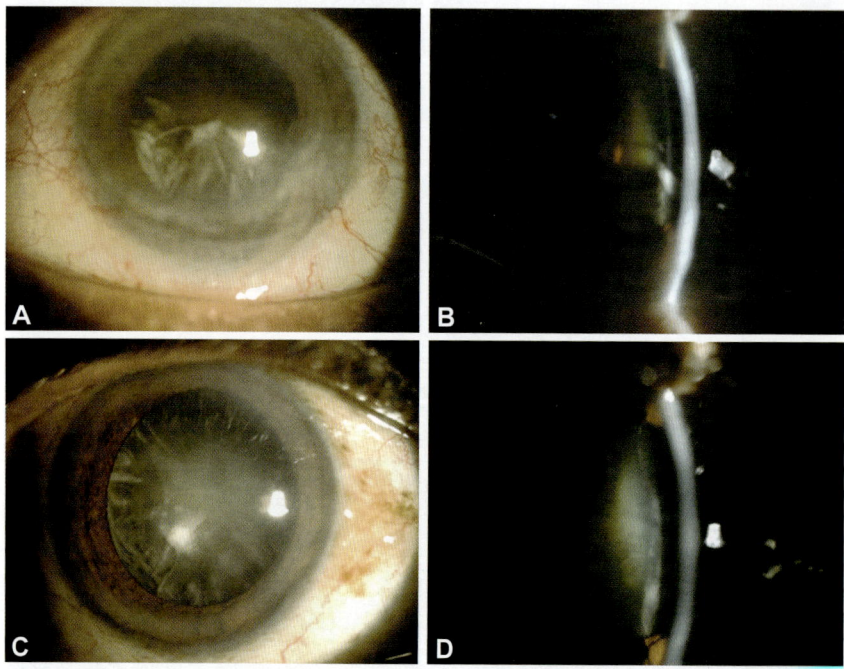

Figs 4A to D (A, C) Gross view, (B, D) Slit view

CORTICAL CATARACT WITH GRADE 1–2 NUCLEUS (FIGS 5A AND B)

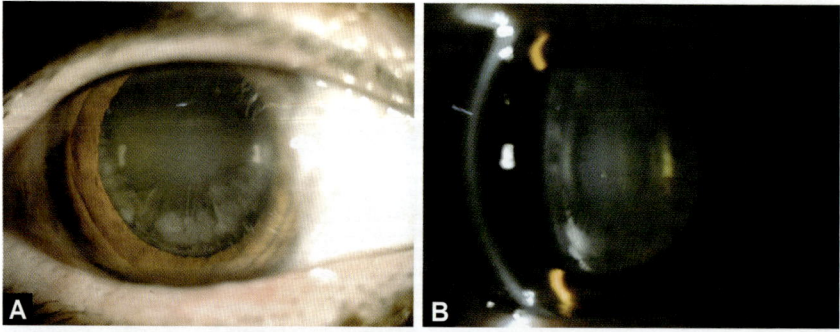

Figs 5A and B (A) Gross view, (B) Slit view

KEY NOTE
Irrigation-aspiration of epinucleus and cortex is always crucial.

Chapter 12

Diffuse Cataract

INTRODUCTION

1. Diffuse means structures of lens are not well demarcated. This is unpredictable variety of cataract. It may be soft or hard and should be tackled accordingly.
2. Phaco surgery is performed as usual depending on the size and hardness of nucleus.
3. Irrigation-aspiration may be difficult as many times tissue is sticky also.

DIFFUSE CATARACT (FIGS 1A AND B)

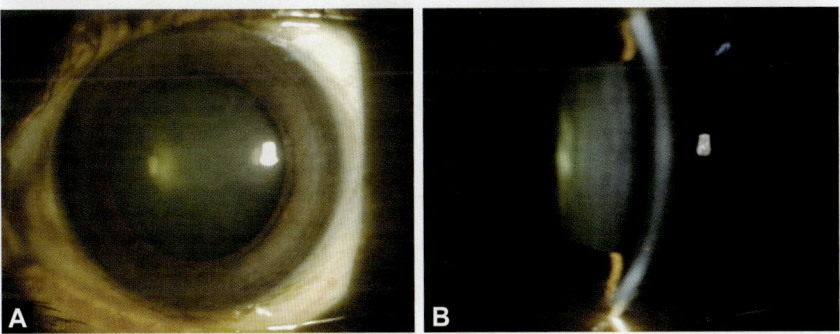

Figs 1A and B (A) Gross view, (B) Slit view

DIFFUSE WITH VERY SOFT NUCLEUS (FIGS 2A AND B)

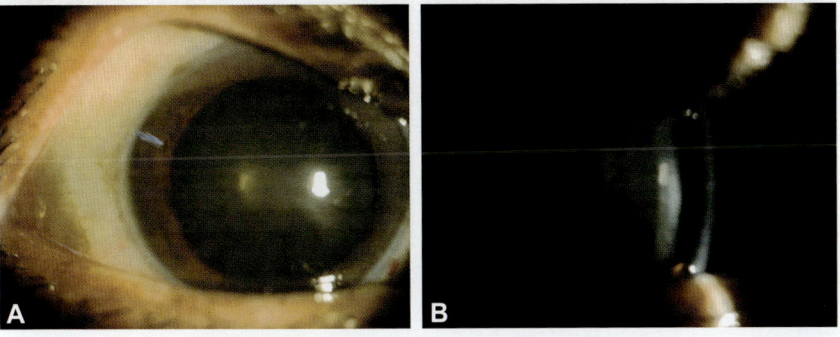

Figs 2A and B (A) Gross view, (B) Slit view

DIFFUSE WITH DEMARCATED NUCLEUS (FIGS 3A AND B)

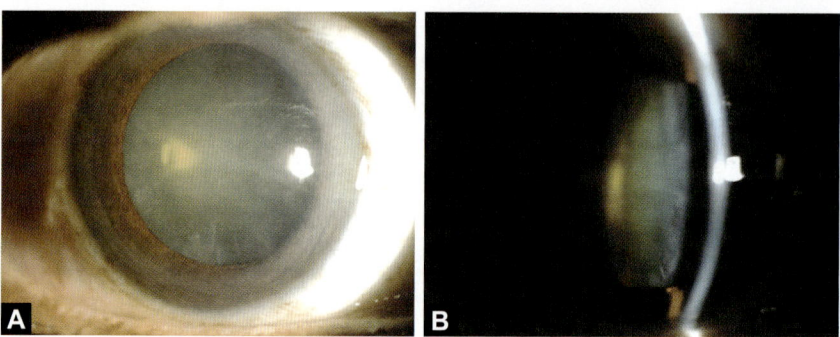

Figs 3A and B (A) Gross view, (B) Slit view

DIFFUSE WITH BIG SIZE NUCLEUS WITH RESPECT TO PUPIL (FIGS 4A AND B)

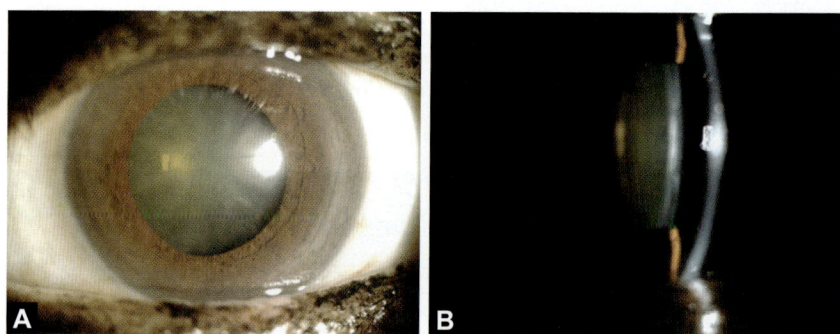

Figs 4A and B (A) Gross view, (B) Slit view

DIFFUSE WITH DENSE NUCLEUS (FIGS 5A AND B)

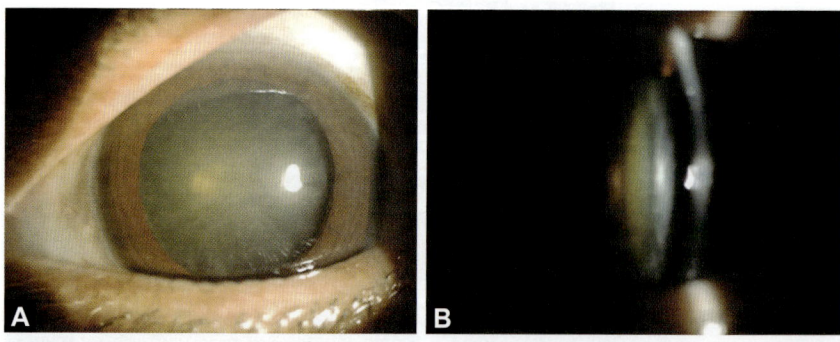

Figs 5A and B (A) Gross view, (B) Slit view

DIFFUSE CATARACT WITH SOFT AND SMALL SIZE NUCLEUS (FIGS 6A AND B)

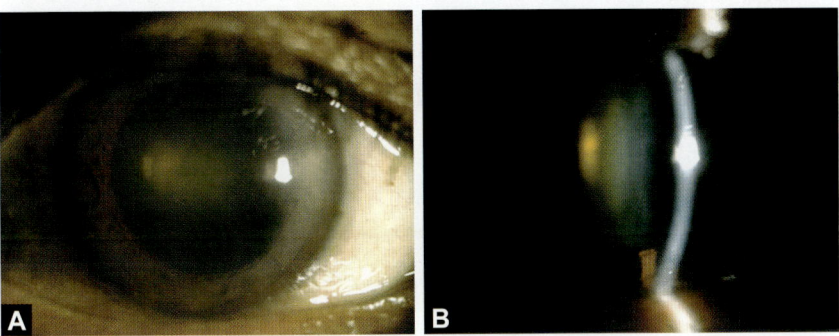

Figs 6A and B (A) Gross view, (B) Slit view

KEY NOTE

Diffuse cataract are usually sticky, hence, irrigation-aspiration of epinucleus and cortex is difficult.

Chapter 13

Cataract with Weak Zone

INTRODUCTION

1. Any opacity in the lens apart from normal site that is nucleus, posterior subcapsular cataract (PSC), anterior subcapsular cataract (ASC) is considered as weak zone in the lens. This is a modified variety of cortical cataract or localized variety of cortical cataract where there is no complete involvement of the cortex but localized to particular segment.
2. *Significance of this variety of cataract is that there is a possibility of zonular weakness in that quadrant. Both eye examination is very important to see the similar opacity in the other eye. This is usually immature variety of cataract.*

CATARACT WITH WEAK ZONE INFERIORLY (FIGS 1A TO F)

Slit Lamp Examination

Gross View

Cataract with weak zone inferiorly.

Slit View

Adequate size and hardness of nucleus.

Advice

1. Easy to do Phaco surgery.
2. Capsulorhexis should be done as usual but inferiorly it should be away from the weak zone.
3. Hydrodelineation can be performed. Minimal or no hydrodissection is required.
4. Direction of strokes of trench should be away from weak zone.
5. In division, avoid undue pressure at inferior part of nucleus.
6. Hold and lift of part of nucleus towards the weak zone should be very slow otherwise there will be traction on zonules.
7. In removal of small pieces, direction of Phaco tip should not be towards the weak zone.

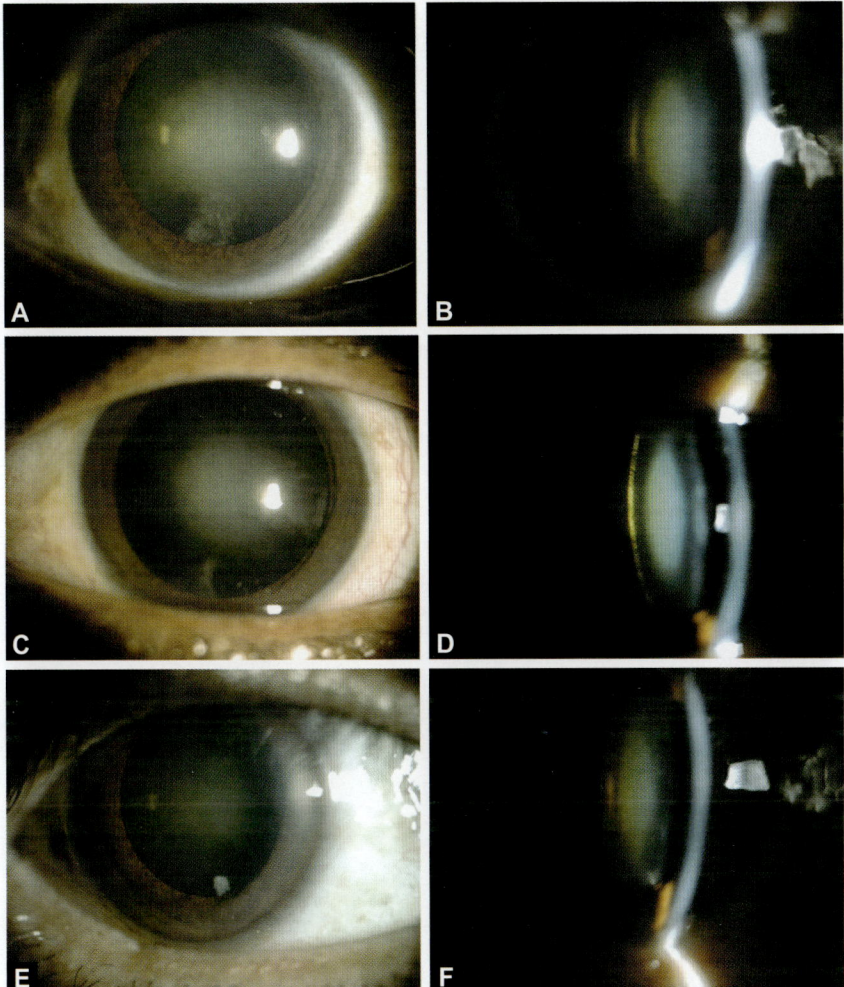

Figs 1A to F (A, C, E) Gross view, (B, D, F) Slit view

8. Irrigation-aspiration of epinucleus and cortex at the weak quadrant should be removed last.
9. In IOL insertion, direction of leading haptic should be away from weak zone, otherwise there may be undue pressure on the bag which may results in zonular dialysis.

CATARACT WITH WEAK ZONE ON SUPERIOR ASPECT (FIGS 2A AND B)

Slit Lamp Examination

Gross View

1. Cataract with weak zone at 12 o'clock.
2. Central small size nuclear cataract.

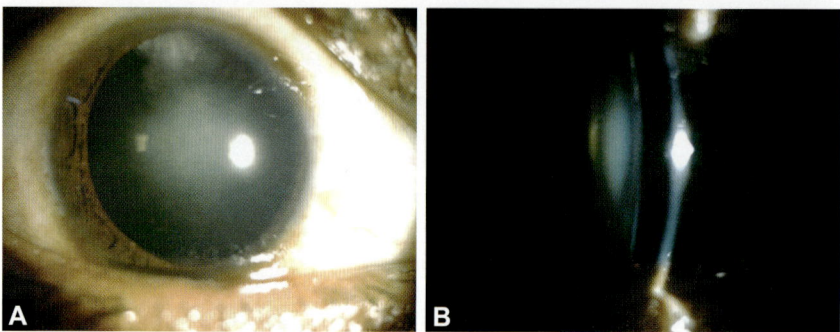

Figs 2A and B (A) Gross view, (B) Slit view

3. Diffuse cortical cataract extending from the superior zone to the central part.

Slit View

Small size of nucleus is confirmed with some element of PSC at the center with element of ASC on the superior aspect.

CATARACT WITH WEAK ZONE FROM 10 TO 1 O'CLOCK POSITION (FIGS 3A AND B)

Slit Lamp Examination

Gross View

Weak zone at 10 to 1 o'clock position.

Slit View

1. Adequate size of nucleus.
2. PSC in central zone.
3. Superiorly opacity seen in cortical area.

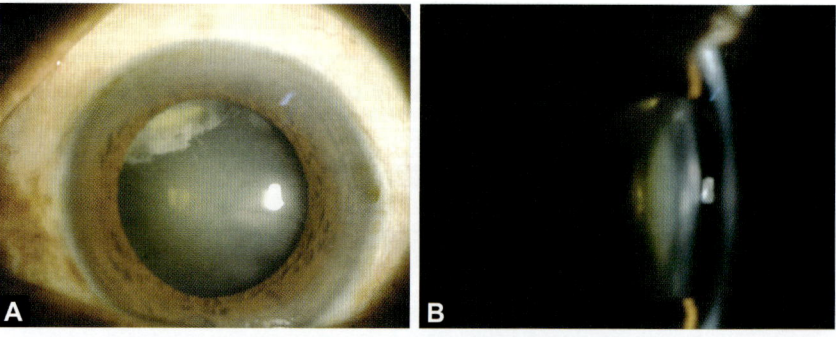

Figs 3A and B (A) Gross view, (B) Slit view

CATARACT WITH WEAK ZONE WITH CENTRAL SMALL NUCLEUS (FIGS 4A AND B)

Slit Lamp Examination

Gross View

Weak zone at 10 to 11 o'clock with central small nucleus.

Slit View

1. Small size nucleus.
2. Grade 2 to 3 dense cataract.

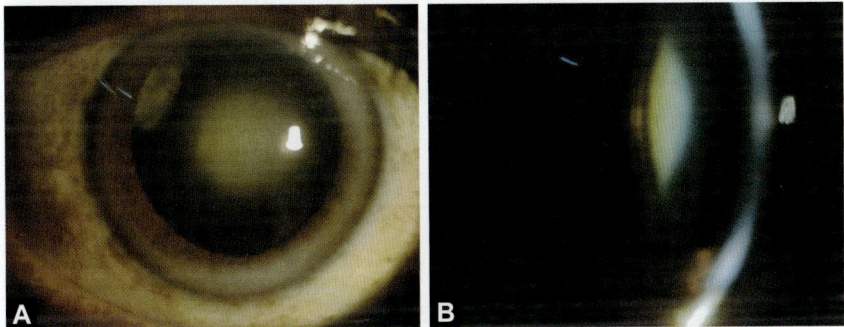

Figs 4A and B (A) Gross view, (B) Slit view

Advice (Figs 2 to 4)

1. Avoid excessive pressure on superior part of nucleus during trench.
2. Avoid pressure superiorly during division and rotation of nucleus.
3. Irrigation-aspiration is difficult and should be done cautiously as it is subincisional.
4. During foldable intraocular lens (IOL) implantation avoid undue pressure superiorly.
5. Passing of the instruments like Phaco tip and irrigation-aspiration cannula through incision and foldable IOL implantation should be gentle as 12 o'clock incision is near the weak zone.

CATARACT WITH WEAK ZONE NASALLY OR TEMPORALLY (FIGS 5A TO E)

Slit Lamp Examination

Gross View (Fig. 5A)

Weak zone from 6 to 11 o'clock.

Gross View (Fig. 5B)

1. Weak zone from 6 to 10 o'clock.
2. Central nuclear cataract.

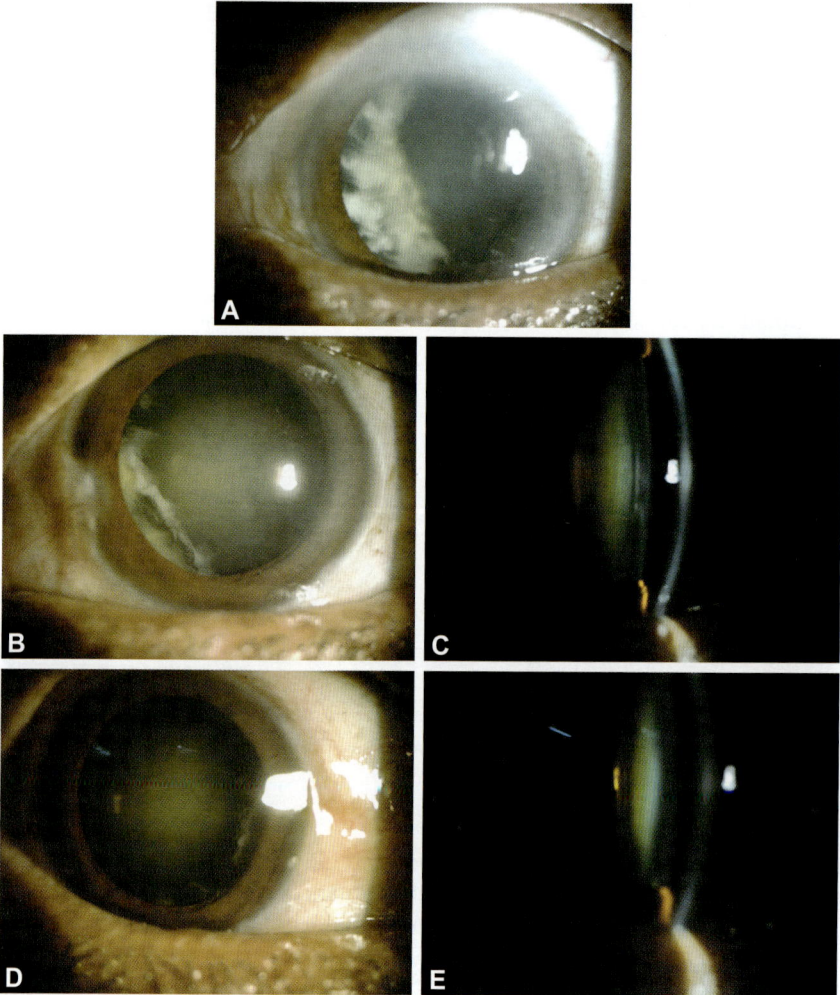

Figs 5A and E (A, B, D) Gross view, (C, E) Slit view

Slit View (Fig. 5C)

1. Adequate size of nucleus.
2. Grade 2 nuclear sclerosis.

Gross View (Fig. 5D)

1. Weak zone from 3 to 6 o'clock.
2. Central nuclear cataract.

Slit View (Fig. 5E)

1. Grade 2 nucleus.
2. Adequate size.

Advice (Figs 5A to E)

1. Phaco surgery is easy.
2. Capsulorhexis should be away from the weak zone.
3. Trench is as usual.
4. In division, no undue pressure on either side.
5. Hold and lift towards the weak zone area should be very slow to avoid pull on the bag which may lead to zonular dehiscence.
6. Irrigation-aspiration should be done at last in the weak zone and should be done tangentially to avoid stretch on zonules.

CATARACT WITH MULTIPLE WEAK ZONES (FIGS 6A AND B)

Slit Lamp Examination

Gross View

Central nuclear cataract with multiple weak zones at the level of cortex.

Slit View

1. Grade 2 nucleus, big size.
2. PSC present, element of ASC confirmed by shadow of ASC on nucleus.

Advice

1. All steps of Phaco surgery should be done cautiously due to multiple weak zones.
2. Capsulorhexis should be away from weak zone.
3. Trench is as usual.
4. In division, no undue pressure on either side.
5. Hold and lift towards the weak zone area should be very slow to avoid pull on the bag which may lead to zonular dehiscence.
6. Irrigation-aspiration should be done at last in the weak zone and should be done tangentially to avoid stretch on zonules.

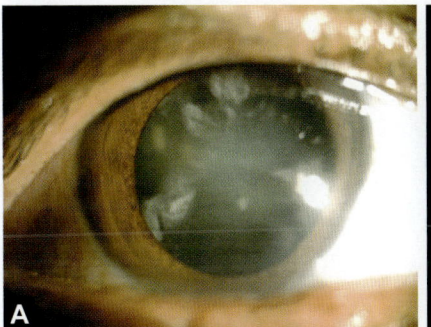 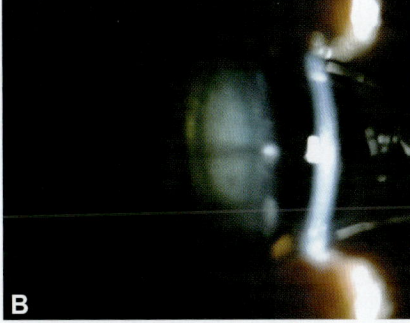

Figs 6A and B (A) Gross view, (B) Slit view

CATARACT WITH WEAK ZONE IN CENTRAL AREA (FIG. 7)

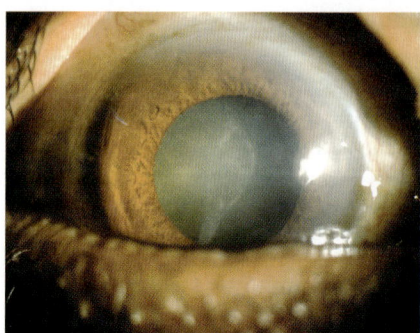

Fig. 7 Gross view

KEY NOTE
1. *Cataract with these considered weak zones should not be taken casual.*
2. *Irrigation-aspiration is always crucial at this site.*

Section 2

Types of Cataract According to Etiology

- Developmental Cataract
- Diabetic Cataract
- Steroid-induced Cataract
- Traumatic Cataract
- Cataract with Uveitis
- Subluxated Cataract

Chapter 14

Developmental Cataract

INTRODUCTION

1. This condition is usually noticed in young patients.
2. Cataract occurs during different stages of development of the lens and type of cataract depends upon that particular developmental stage of lens.
3. This is the soft variety of cataract.

Advice

1. Cataract extraction has to be done as early as possible to prevent amblyopia.
2. Capsulorhexis is difficult. High molecular weight viscoelastic agents may be needed.
3. Hydrodissection has to be done.
4. Viscoexpression of the lens matter is unique way to remove the cataract. Hydrophobic foldable intraocular lens (IOL) is the lens of choice. In some cases primary posterior capsulotomy with anterior vitrectomy may be needed.

DIFFERENT VARIETY OF DEVELOPMENTAL CATARACT (FIGS 1 TO 7)

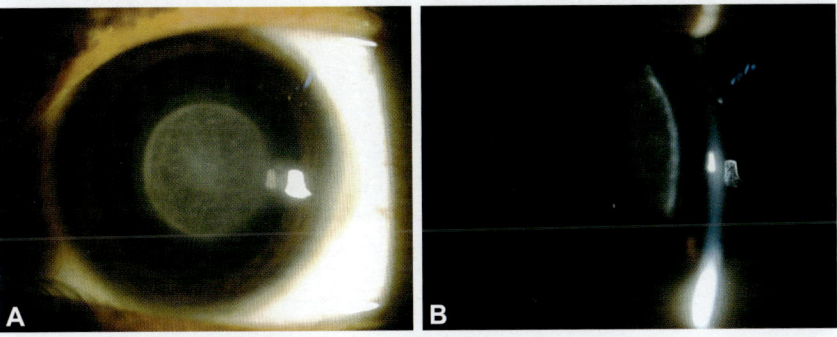

Figs 1A and B (A) Gross view, (B) Slit view

78 Section 2: Types of Cataract According to Etiology

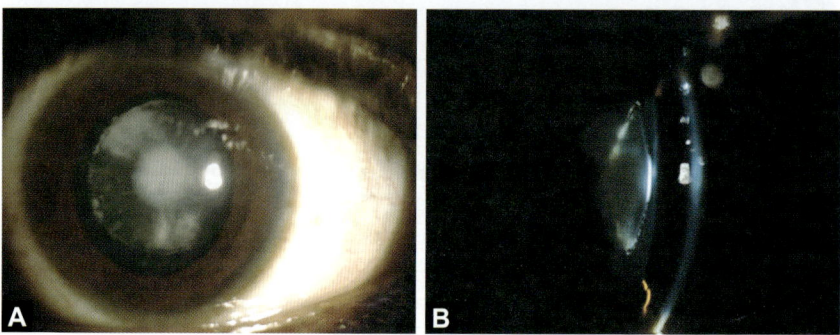

Figs 2A and B (A) Gross view, (B) Slit view

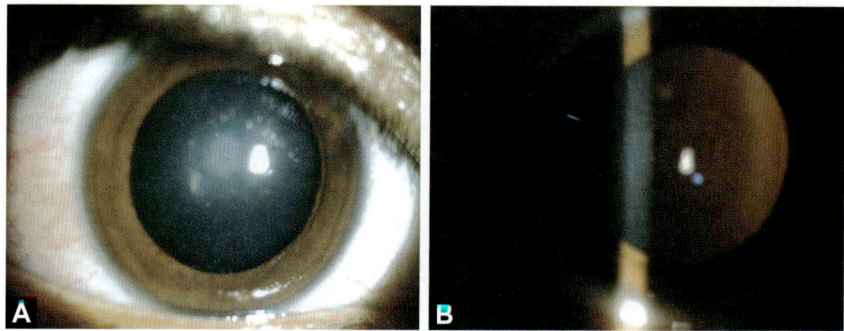

Figs 3A and B (A) Gross view, (B) Slit view

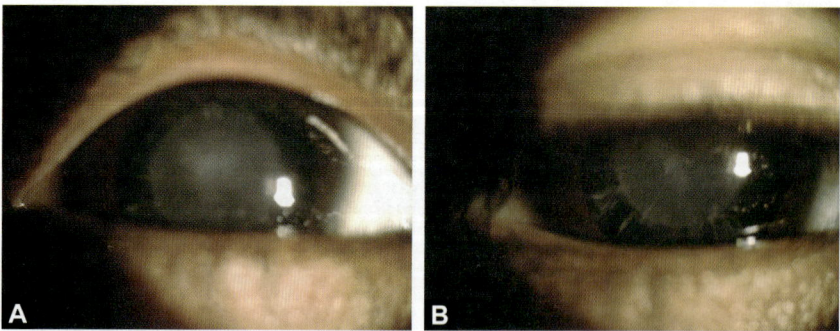

Figs 4A and B (A) Gross view, (B) Slit view

Chapter 14: Developmental Cataract

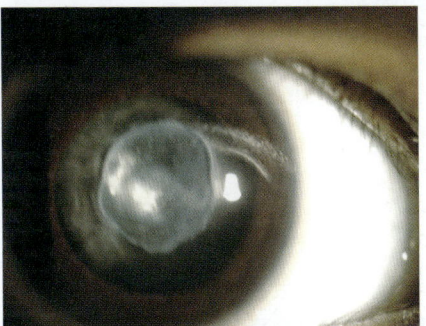

Fig. 5 Gross view

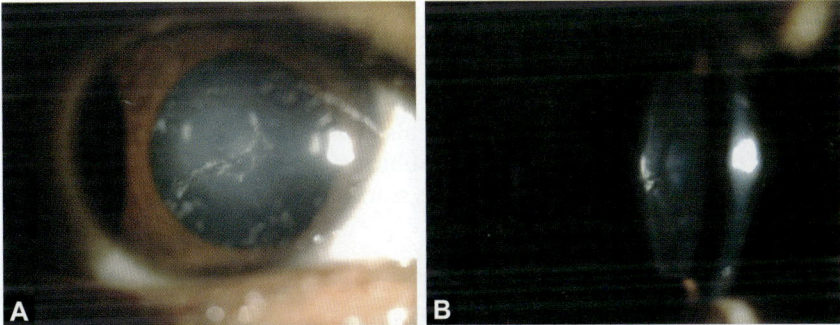

Figs 6A and B (A) Gross view, (B) Slit view

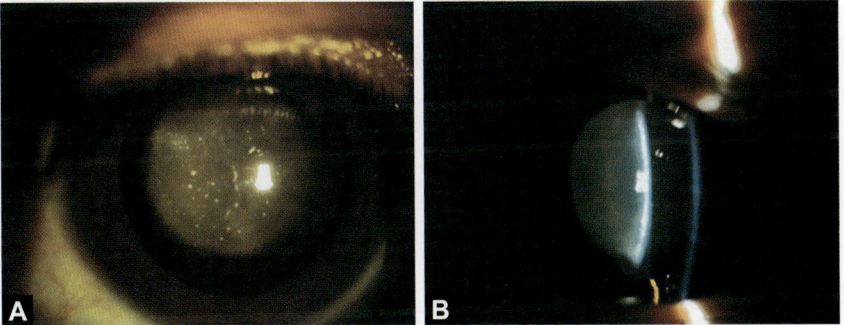

Figs 7A and B (A) Gross view, (B) Slit view

KEY NOTE
Capsulorhexis is the most difficult step in these cases.

Chapter 15

Diabetic Cataract

INTRODUCTION

1. Cataract and diabetes has unique correlation with each other.
2. Cataract can be immature, mature, hypermature or hard variety.
3. These cataracts occur at early age also. Location of cataract varies from case to case. It can be anterior subcapsular cataract (ASC), posterior subcapsular cataract (PSC), diffuse, soft, hard, brown, sticky, swollen lens and cortical variety.

Advice

Phaco surgery depends on the type of cataract and anatomy of the eye.

TYPICAL DIABETIC CATARACT (FIGS 1A TO C)

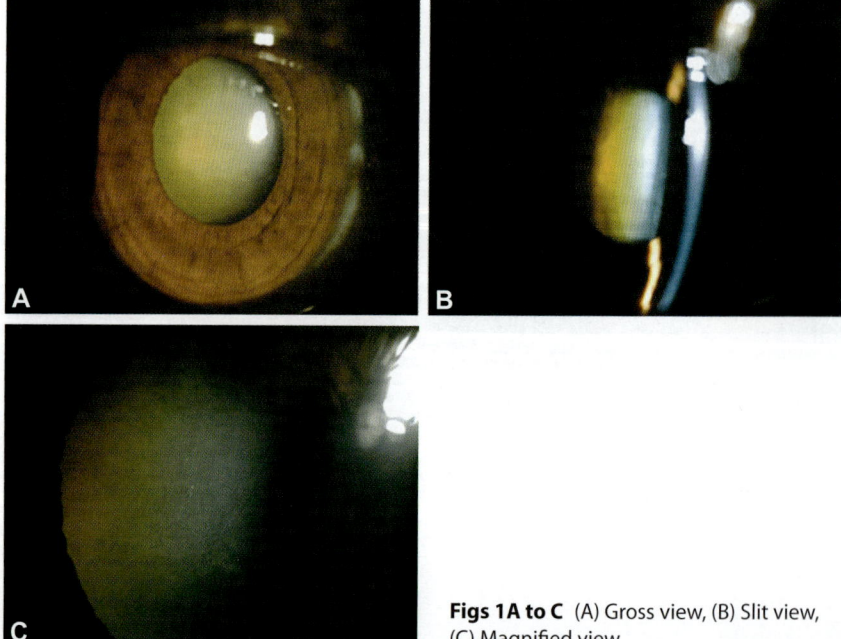

Figs 1A to C (A) Gross view, (B) Slit view, (C) Magnified view

Slit Lamp Examination

Gross View

1. Dense cataract.
2. Undilated pupil.

Slit View

1. All layers of the lens are seen.
2. Big size (bulky) nucleus.
3. Dense posterior subcapsular cataract also seen.

MATURE CATARACT (FIGS 2A AND B)

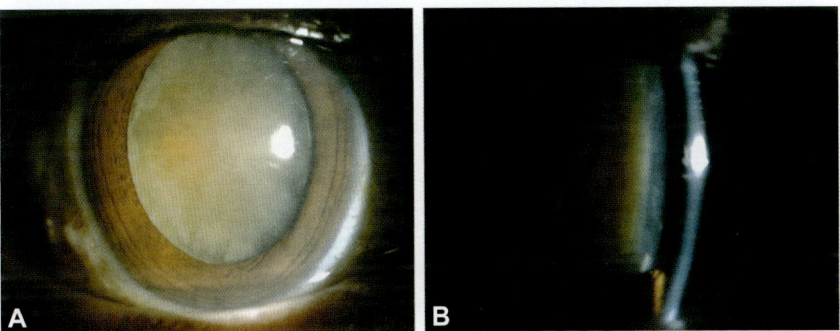

Figs 2A and B (A) Gross view, (B) Slit view

Slit Lamp Examination

Gross View

1. Mature cataract.
2. Dilated pupil.

Slit View

1. All layers of the lens are seen.
2. Hard and brown cataract, (grade 4 to 5 dense nucleus) big bulky nucleus.
3. Thick sheet of epinucleus.

SOFT CATARACT (FIGS 3A AND B)

Slit Lamp Examination

Gross View

1. Immature cataract.
2. Dilated pupil.

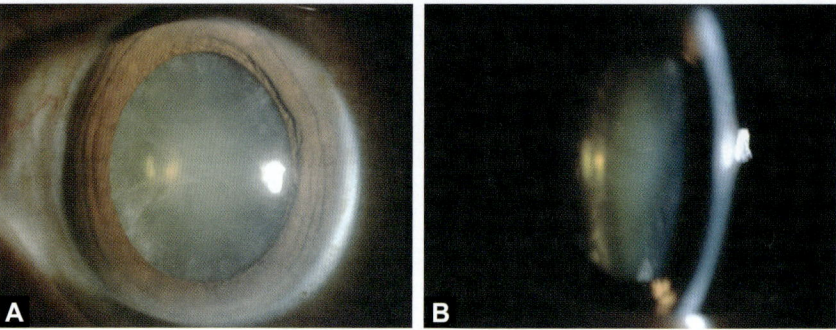

Figs 3A and B (A) Gross view, (B) Slit view

Slit View

1. All layers of the lens could be seen.
2. Soft and bulky nucleus.
3. Thick sheet of epinucleus all around nucleus is visible.

CORTICAL AND DIFFUSE CATARACT (FIGS 4A AND B)

Slit Lamp Examination

Gross View

Cortical and diffuse cataract.

Slit View

1. All layers of the lens could be seen.
2. Cortical elements are seen as a shadow on the nucleus.
3. Big and bulky nucleus but soft.

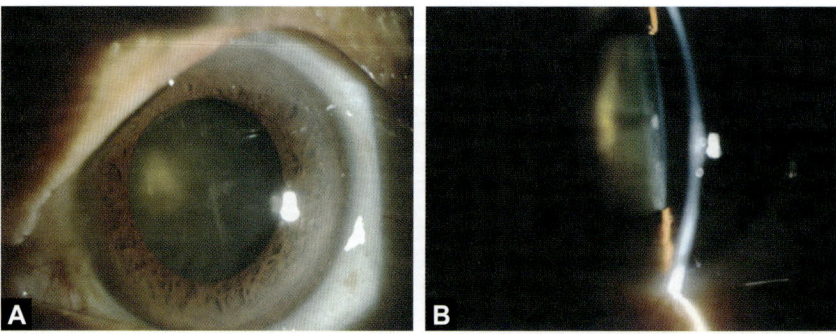

Figs 4A and B (A) Gross view, (B) Slit view

Chapter 15: Diabetic Cataract

VERY SOFT CATARACT (FIGS 5A AND B)

Slit Lamp Examination

Gross View

1. Immature cataract.
2. Cortical component is seen.

Slit View

1. All layers of the lens are seen.
2. Centrally empty space is labeled as bulky soft tissue with no hardness (no nucleus).
3. Thick sheet of epinucleus.

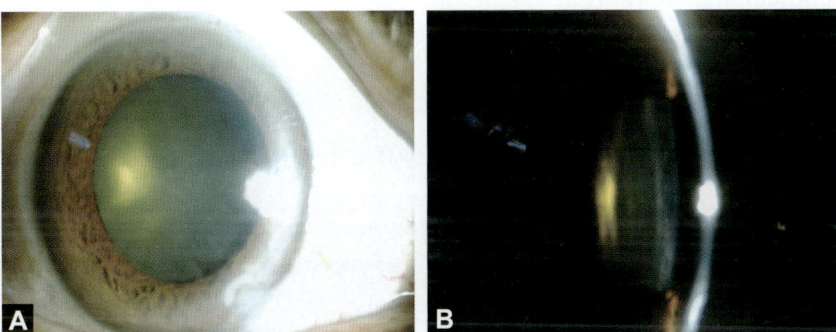

Figs 5A and B (A) Gross view, (B) Slit view

CENTRAL ANTERIOR SUBCAPSULAR CATARACT (FIGS 6A AND B)

Slit Lamp Examination

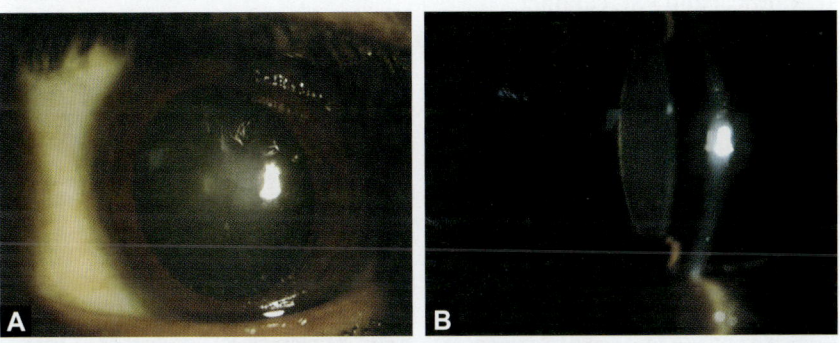

Figs 6A and B (A) Gross view, (B) Slit view

Gross View

1. Immature cataract.
2. Central ASC.

Slit View

1. Soft cataract.
2. ASC and PSC is also noted.

CORTICAL CATARACT (FIGS 7A AND B)

Slit Lamp Examination

Gross View

Cortical cataract is seen in magnified view which is confirmed by retroillumination view.

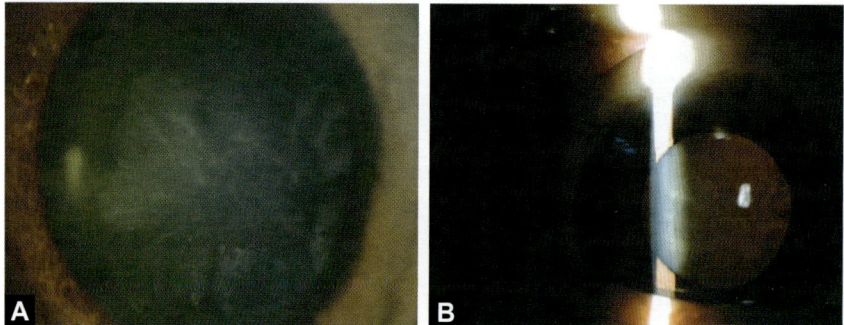

Figs 7A and B (A) Magnified view, (B) Retroillumination view

DIFFERENT VARIETY OF CORTICAL CATARACT (FIGS 8A AND B)

Slit Lamp Examination

Gross View

1. Cortical and PSC cataract.
2. Retroillumination shows droplet variety of PSC is typical in diabetic cases.

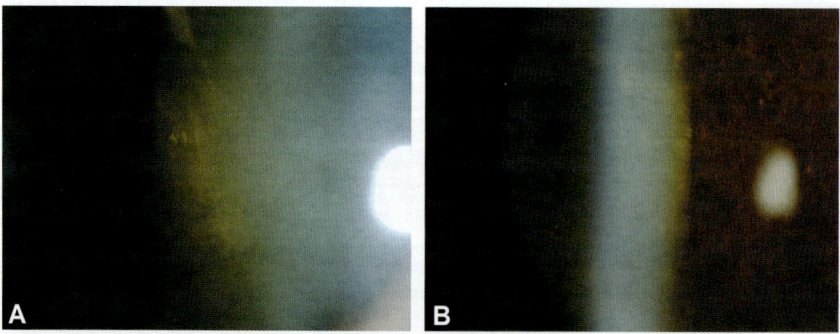

Figs 8A and B (A) Gross view, (B) Retroillumination view

CATARACT WITH NEOVASCULAR GLAUCOMA (FIG. 9)

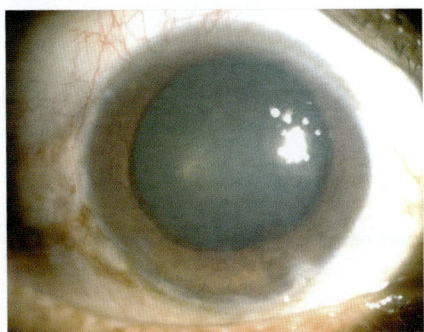

Fig. 9 Cataract with neovascular glaucoma

Slit Lamp Examination

Gross View

Cataract with neovascular glaucoma and ectropion uveae.
It means that in every diabetic cases iris has to be examined in detail.

KEY NOTE
1. *Diabetic cataract present with different varities.*
2. *Morphologically we have noticed bulky nucleus and sticky component of cataract in many cases.*

Chapter 16

Steroid-induced Cataract

INTRODUCTION

1. Cataract is due to use of steroid for a longer period. It is not only systemic steroids but also local steroids in the form of drops, ointment, injectable can induce cataract.
2. This variety of cataract is generally seen in young patients.
3. It is a soft variety of cataract, usually posterior subcapsular.
4. Phaco surgery is performed as in a soft cataract.

POSTERIOR SUBCAPSULAR CATARACT (FIGS 1A AND B)

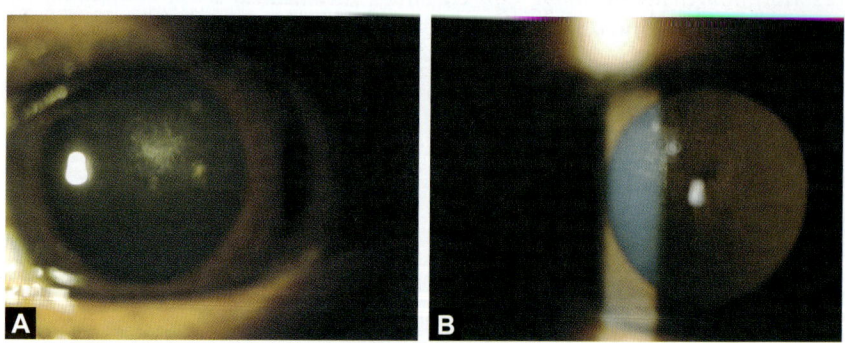

Figs 1A and B (A) Gross view, (B) Retroillumination view

Slit Lamp Examination

Gross View

1. Posterior subcapsular cataract (PSC) is confirmed on retroillumination.
2. This is a typical variety of steroid induced cataract.

DENSE POSTERIOR SUBCAPSULAR CATARACT (FIGS 2A AND B)

Slit Lamp Examination

Gross View

Dense posterior subcapsular cataract.

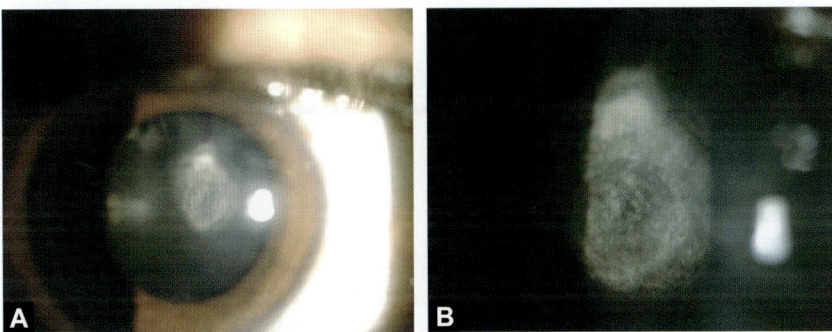

Figs 2A and B (A) Gross view, (B) Magnified view

DIFFUSE CATARACT (FIGS 3A AND B)

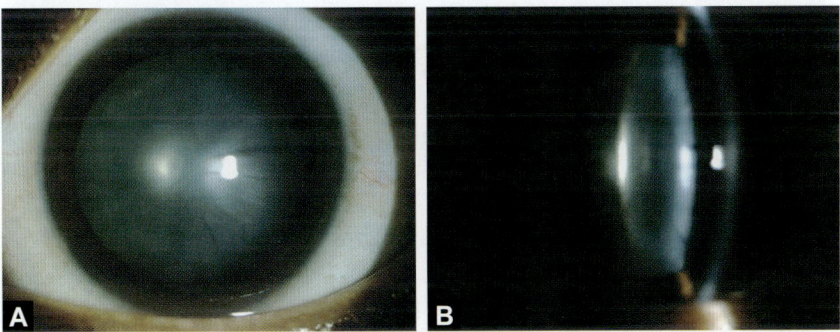

Figs 3A and B (A) Gross view, (B) Slit view

Slit Lamp Examination

Gross View

Diffuse cataract.

Slit View

1. Soft nucleus.
2. Cortical and central posterior subcapsular cataract.

KEY NOTE
Steroid-induced cataract is usually a soft cataract and management is as in cases of soft cataract.

Chapter 17

Traumatic Cataract

INTRODUCTION

1. Traumatic cataract occurs secondary to trauma.
2. Two common ways of trauma are blunt and penetrating. Due to blunt trauma, traumatic cataract is frequently associated with the zonular dehiscence. In penetrating injury usually there can be injury to the lens structure and cataract can occur to any layer of the lens.
3. In this chapter, we are mainly considering the photographs of traumatic cataract which are treatable. Cases due to blunt trauma presented as subluxated cataract will be described later.
4. *Management of traumatic cataract varies from case to case.*

DIFFUSE CATARACT WITH POSTERIOR SYNECHIAE (FIGS 1A AND B)

Slit Lamp Examination

Gross View

Diffuse cataract with posterior synechiae.

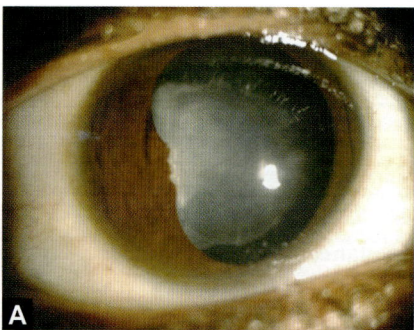 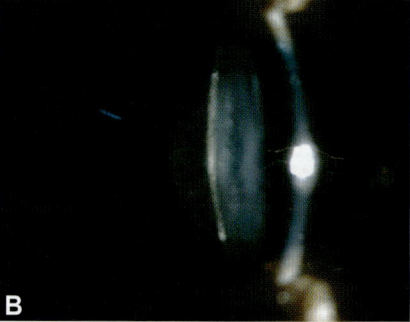

Figs 1A and B (A) Gross view, (B) Slit view

Slit View

1. All layers of the lens are well defined.
2. Diffuse cataract is confirmed.

Advice

1. Management is easy in this case which can be done through Phaco surgery incision.
2. Incision should be limbal.
3. *Do not break the posterior synechiae which give good support to the capsular bag. This is one of the important points of consideration in the management of these cases.*
4. Capsulorhexis can be done easily which should be away from posterior synechiae.
5. Gentle hydroprocedure or viscodelineation is needed.
6. Irrigation-aspiration of soft lens material can be easily done.
7. Foldable intraocular lens (IOL) implantation can be done.

CATARACT WITH CENTRAL POSTERIOR SYNECHIAE (FIGS 2A AND B)

Slit Lamp Examination

Gross View

1. Iris pigment on the lens.
2. Pupil is not fully dilated because of central dense posterior synechiae.

Slit View

1. Corneal scar is seen which is secondary to trauma.
2. Convexity of the iris is noticed inferiorly which may indicate lens material pushing the iris forward.

Advice

This case is not very easy as there is localized injury to the capsule inferiorly where iris bulging is seen. Exact condition of the lens cannot be seen as it is hidden behind the iris. There are always chances of PCR during surgery.

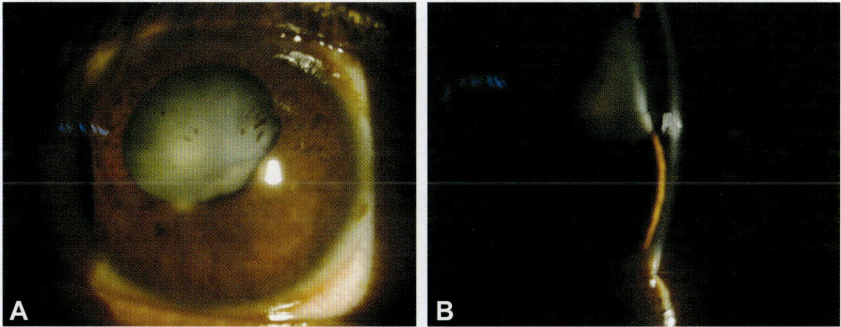

Figs 2A and B (A) Gross view, (B) Slit view

ANTERIOR CAPSULAR CATARACT (FIG. 3)

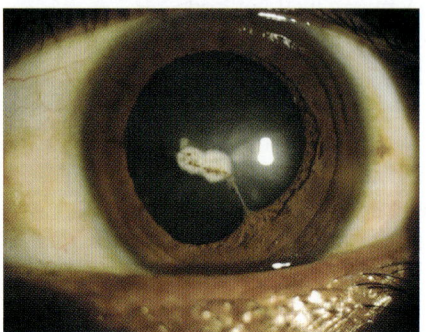

Fig. 3 Gross view

Slit Lamp Examination

Gross View

Localized anterior capsular lesion with iris band attached.

Advice

It is not very difficult case as tissue damage is localized to central zone.
1. Pupil is adequately dilated.
2. Cut the iris band. The part of anterior capsule removed by capsulorhexis should include that lesion. Rest of the nucleus management is according to the density of nucleus.
3. Possibility of posterior capsule rupture (PCR) is there during surgery.

TRAUMATIC CATARACT WITH RUPTURE OF ANTERIOR CAPSULE (FIGS 4A TO D)

Slit Lamp Examination

Gross View

1. Traumatic cataract with rupture of anterior capsule from 12 to 6 o'clock. Which is clearly seen on magnified view.
2. Iris pigment at the cornea indicates injury through cornea and iris.

Advice

1. It is a soft cataract.
2. Crucial part in this case is management of the capsule. Capsulotomy with Vanna's scissor can be done to relax the capsule and then can be completed with the help of microcapsulorhexis forceps.
3. Manual aspiration of the soft tissue with Simcoe cannula should be done followed by foldable IOL implantation.

Chapter 17: Traumatic Cataract

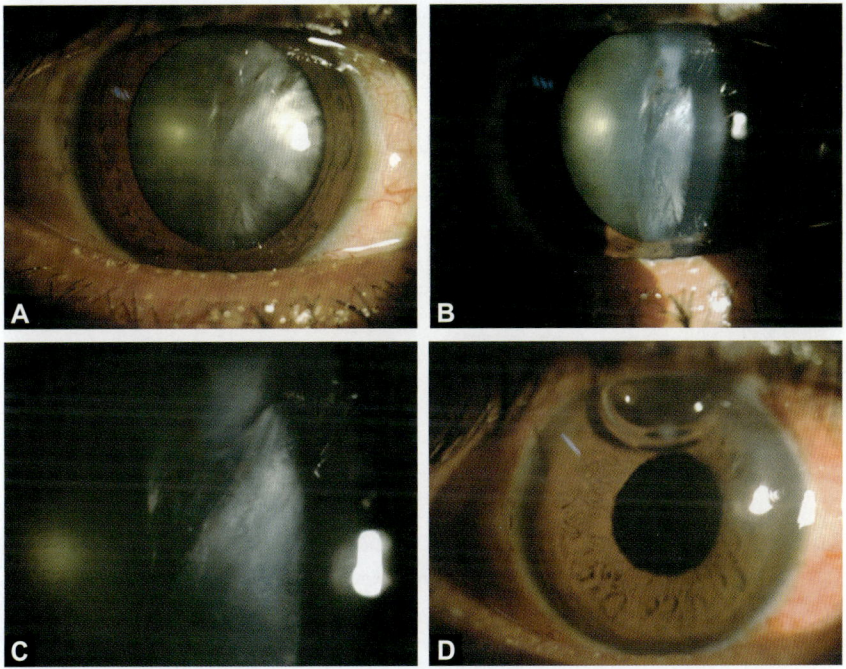

Figs 4A to D (A, B) Gross view, (C) Magnified, (D) Postoperative view

TRAUMATIC CATARACT WITH ANTERIOR CAPSULE RUPTURE (FIG. 5)

Slit Lamp Examination

Gross View

1. Traumatic cataract with anterior capsule rupture. Lens material has popped out of the bag and some soft tissue material has seen dispersed

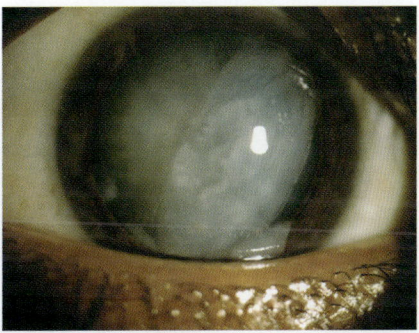

Fig. 5 Gross view rupture of anterior capsule with lens material in anterior chamber

in anterior chamber. Sometimes, it is an important sign in trauma cases which indirectly indicates that posterior capsule may be intact.
2. Management as mentioned earlier.

TRAUMATIC ANTERIOR SUBCAPSULAR CATARACT (FIGS 6A AND B)

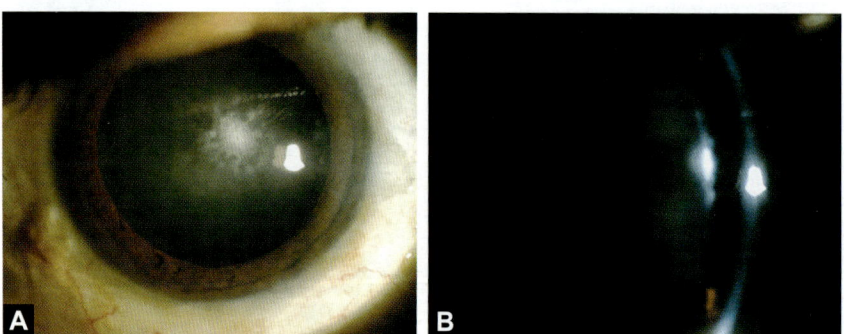

Figs 6A and B (A) Gross view, (B) Slit view

Slit Lamp Examination

Gross View

Traumatic anterior subcapsular cataract (ASC).

Slit View

Anterior subcapsular cataract with soft nuclear cataract.

TRAUMATIC DIFFUSE ANTERIOR SUBCAPSULAR CATARACT (FIGS 7A AND B)

Slit Lamp Examination

Gross View

Traumatic ASC which is widely spread.

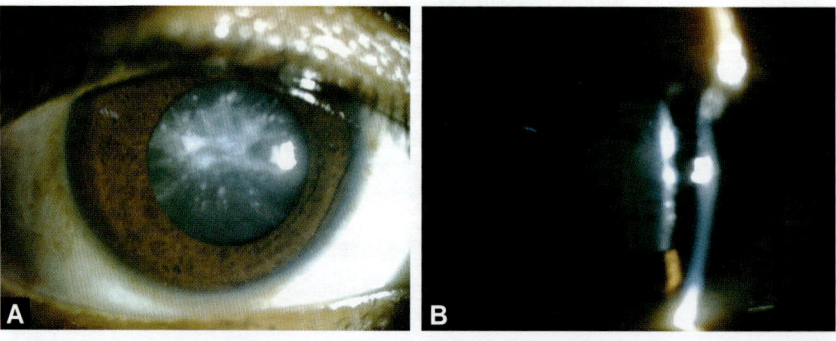

Figs 7A and B (A) Gross view, (B) Slit view

Slit View

ASC with soft nuclear cataract.

Advice (Figs 6 and 7)

1. Try to include this lesion within the boundary of capsulorhexis which is easily possible in localized ASC.
2. Rest of the management as if in soft cataract.

ADHERENT LEUKOMA WITH POSTERIOR SYNECHIAE (FIG. 8)

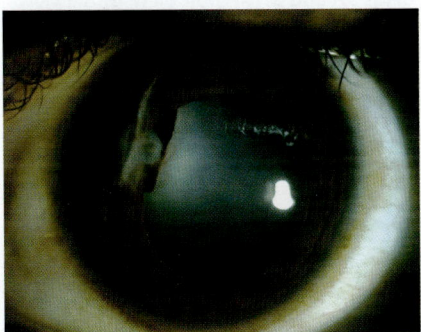

Fig. 8 Gross view

Slit Lamp Examination

Gross View

Linear corneal scar, adherent leukoma with posterior synechiae. It means that the cornea, iris and capsular bag are adhering to each other.

Advice

1. *Do not break anterior and posterior synechiae.*
2. Capsulorhexis is important and possible.
3. Rest of the management is easy in this case.

TRAUMATIC NEARLY MATURE CATARACT WITH POSTERIOR SYNECHIAE (FIGS 9A AND B)

Slit Lamp Examination

Gross View

1. Traumatic nearly mature cataract with posterior synechiae.
2. Pupil is not fully dilated.

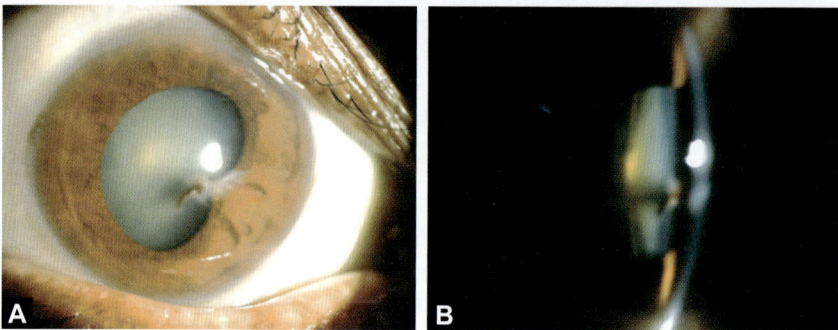

Figs 9A and B (A) Gross view, (B) Slit view

Slit View

1. Site of injury on the cornea, iris and lens is confirmed.
2. Adequate density and size of the nucleus.

Advice

Phaco surgery is advisable.

TRAUMATIC CATARACT WITH IRIDODIALYSIS (FIGS 10A AND B)

Slit Lamp Examination

Gross View

Traumatic cataract with iridodialysis more than 180 degrees.

Advice

1. This case is difficult to treat.
2. In these cases, iridodialysis and traumatic cataract should be managed.

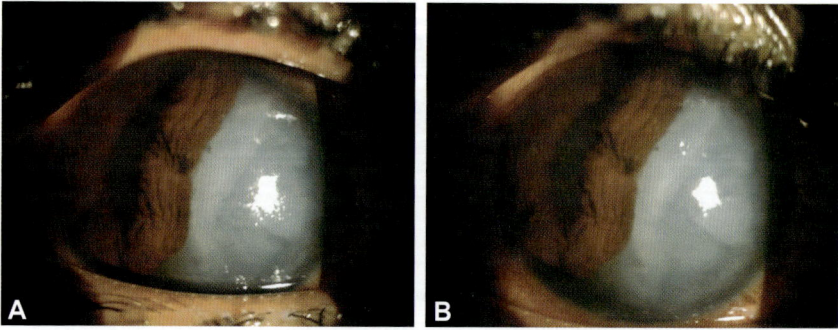

Figs 10A and B Gross view

TRAUMATIC CATARACT WITH LOCALIZED IRIDODIALYSIS (FIGS 11A AND B)

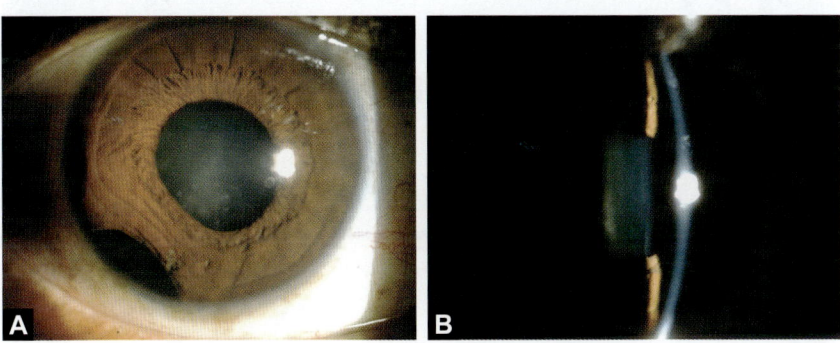

Figs 11A and B (A) Gross view, (B) Slit view

Slit Lamp Examination

Gross View

Traumatic cataract with localized iridodialysis at 7 o'clock position.

Slit View

Soft cataract.

Advice

Relatively easy to treat.

KEY NOTE
Presentation of traumatic cataract is deferred from case-to-case. So the management varies.

Chapter 18

Cataract with Uveitis

INTRODUCTION

1. In this situation pupil is small, due to eye inflammation, all the anatomy of the eye is deranged and compromised.
2. Cataract surgery has to be done under the cover of steroids.
3. High molecular weight viscoelastic agents are needed to protect the cornea, and to maintain the dilatation of the pupil.
4. All the necessary management related to small pupil is needed.
5. Phaco surgery is possible in immature cataract. In very hard and mature cataract, one can think of doing SICS/ECCE.

IMMATURE CATARACT WITH POSTERIOR SYNECHIAE (FIGS 1A AND B)

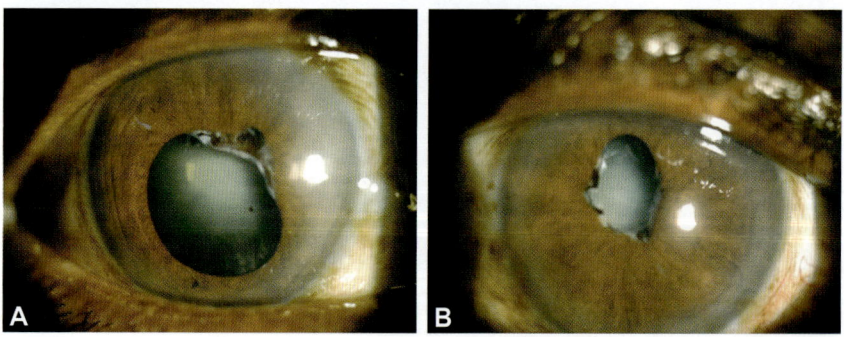

Figs 1A and B Gross view

Slit Lamp Examination

Gross View

1. Immature cataract
2. Pupil is not fully dilated
3. Adequate size of the nucleus is seen in the center.

Advice

Phaco surgery is possible

HARD CATARACT WITH POSTERIOR SYNECHIAE (FIG. 2)

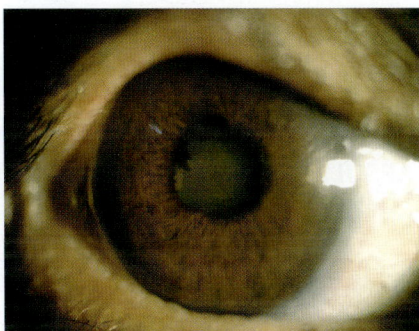

Fig. 2 Gross view

Slit Lamp Examination

Gross View

1. Hard cataract with posterior synechiae
2. Hazy cornea.

Advice

1. Phaco surgery can be done with some modifications as mentioned above with caution
2. Converting to SICS or ECCE may be required.

NEARLY MATURE CATARACT WITH POSTERIOR SYNECHIAE (FIG. 3)

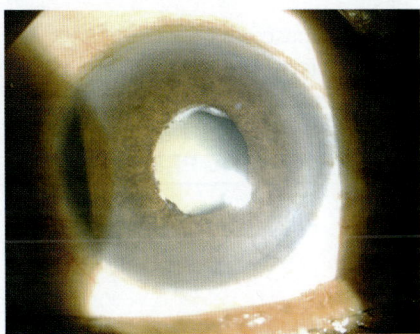

Fig. 3 Gross view

Slit Lamp Examination

Gross View

1. Nearly mature cataract with posterior synechiae
2. Pupil is small.

Advice

Phaco surgery is possible taking in consideration the maturity of the cataract and pupillary size.

POSTERIOR SUBCAPSULAR CATARACT (FIGS 4A AND B)

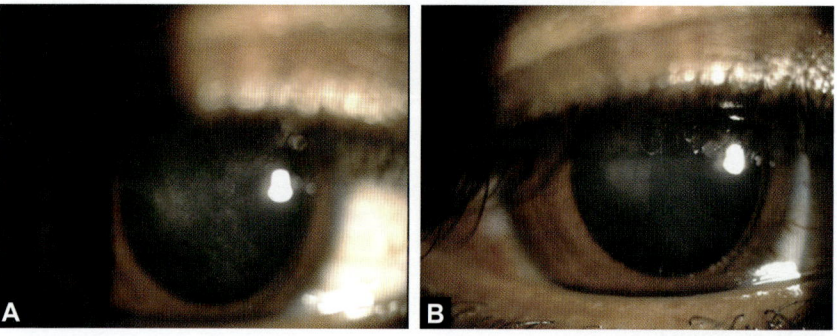

Figs 4A and B Gross view: (A) Posterior subcapsular cataract (light focused on the capsule), (B) Keratic precipitates are seen on the cornea (light focused on the cornea)

Slit Lamp Examination

Gross View

PSC with keratic precipitates.

Advice

1. Phaco surgery is easy
2. All management is like in case of PSC
3. High molecular weight viscoelastic agents are essential which coats the endothelium to protect cornea during surgery.

DIFFUSE CATARACT WITH KERATIC PRECIPITATES (FIGS 5A TO C)

Slit Lamp Examination

Gross View

1. Diffuse cataract with keratic precipitates
2. Dilated pupil.

Slit View

1. All layers of the lens are seen
2. Diffuse cataract is confirmed
3. It is soft cataract.

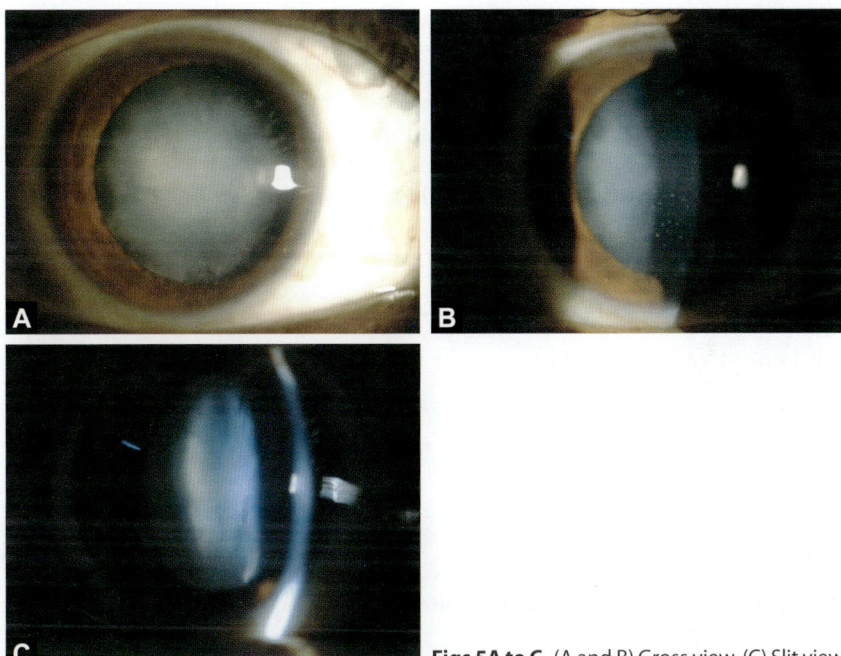

Figs 5A to C (A and B) Gross view, (C) Slit view

Advice

Phaco surgery is easy.

MATURE CATARACT WITH POSTERIOR SYNECHIAE (FIG. 6)

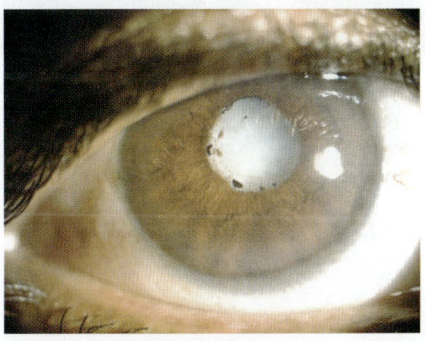

Fig. 6 Gross view

Slit Lamp Examination

Gross View

1. Mature cataract with small pupil
2. Posterior synechiae seen at all around 360 degrees of lens circumference
3. Iris pigment deposition is seen on the anterior capsule.

Advice

1. Management of small pupil is essential
2. Phaco surgery is not very difficult as cornea is clear
3. Sometimes conversion to SICS and ECCE is needed.

FESTOONED SHAPED PUPIL WITH IMMATURE CATARACT (FIGS 7A AND B)

Slit Lamp Examination

Gross View

1. Immature cataract
2. Festoon shaped pupil.

Slit View

Posterior subcapsular cataract is noticed.

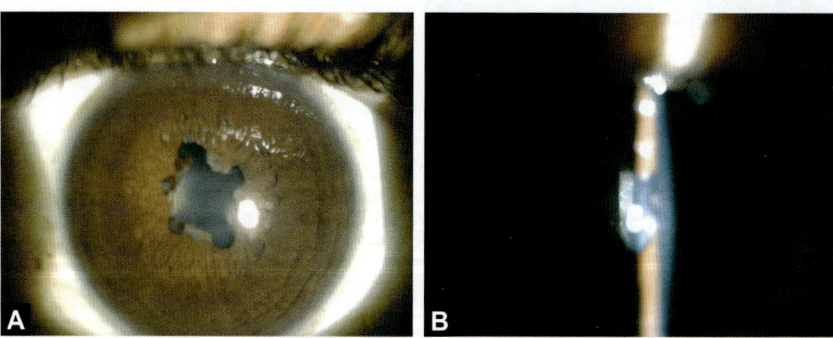

Figs 7A and B (A) Gross view, (B) Slit view

Advice

Phaco surgery is possible after management of pupil.

FESTOONED SHAPED PUPIL WITH MATURE CATARACT (FIG. 8)

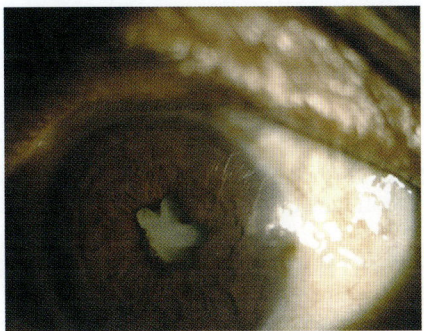

Fig. 8 Gross view

Slit Lamp Examination

Gross View

Festooned shaped pupil with mature cataract.

Advice

1. Phaco surgery is not very easy but possible
2. One can think of converting the case to SICS or ECCE.

ECTROPION UVEAE WITH HARD CATARACT (FIGS 9A AND B)

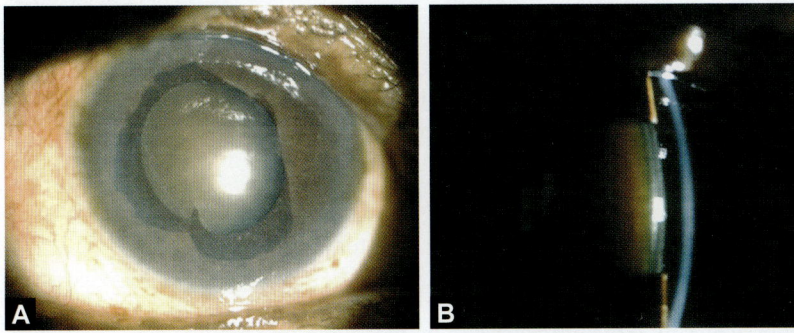

Figs 9A and B (A) Gross view, (B) Slit view

Slit Lamp Examination

Gross View

1. Ectropion uveae with hard cataract
2. Semidilated pupil.

Slit View

1. All layers of the lens are seen
2. Grade 4 to 5 dense nucleus
3. Long length of nucleus as both edges of nucleus hide behind the pupil.

Advice

1. Phaco surgery is not very easy
2. The surgeon can seen face difficulty during SICS or ECCE.

MATURE CATARACT WITH PATCHES OF IRIS ATROPHY AND POSTERIOR SYNECHIAE (FIG. 10)

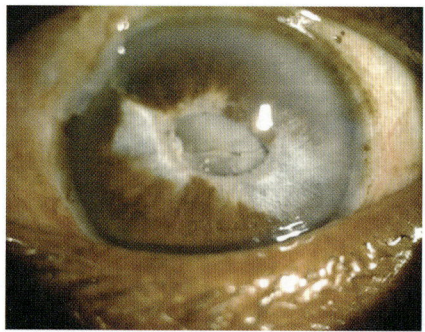

Fig. 10 Gross view

Slit Lamp Examination

Gross View

1. Mature cataract with posterior synechiae
2. Patches of iris atrophy with loss of iris pattern
3. Filtering bleb is seen at 10 o'clock position.

Advice

As it is very complicated case, ECCE is a better choice.

KEY NOTE

It is a very complicated cataract can be managed under full cover of steroids. Small pupil management is the most important factor in this situation.

Chapter 19

Subluxated Cataract

INTRODUCTION

1. By definition, cataractous lens displaced partially from the pupillary area is called as subluxation of cataract. This subluxation is due to zonular weakness.
2. Etiology is congenital and acquired. Acquired causes can be trauma, mature cataract, hypermature cataract, old age, very hard cataract, advanced pseudoexfoliation etc.
3. Management of subluxated cataract varies from case to case and can be managed by Phaco surgery, small incision cataract surgery (SICS) or extracapsular cataract extraction (ECCE).
4. Assistant tools are capsular tension ring (CTR), CTR injector, iris hook, capsular hooks, modified CTR, prolene suture, scleral fixation intraocular lens (IOL), iris claw IOL, glued IOL, anterior chamber IOL, high viscocity viscoelastic agent, and vitrectomy unit.

HYPERMATURE CATARACT WITH INFERIOR SUBLUXATION (FIGS 1A AND B)

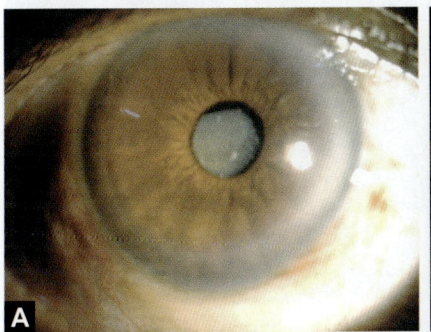
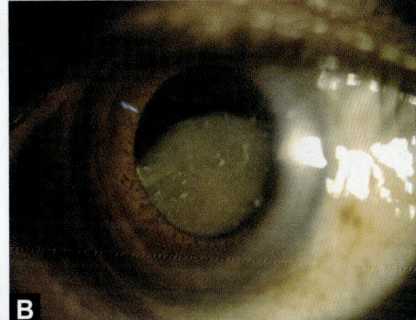

Figs 1A and B Gross view

Slit Lamp Examination

Gross View

1. Hypermature sclerotic cataract.
2. Inferior subluxation 180 degrees.

HYPERMATURE CATARACT WITH INFERIOR SUBLUXATION AND CALCIFIED CAPSULAR BAG (FIGS 2A AND B)

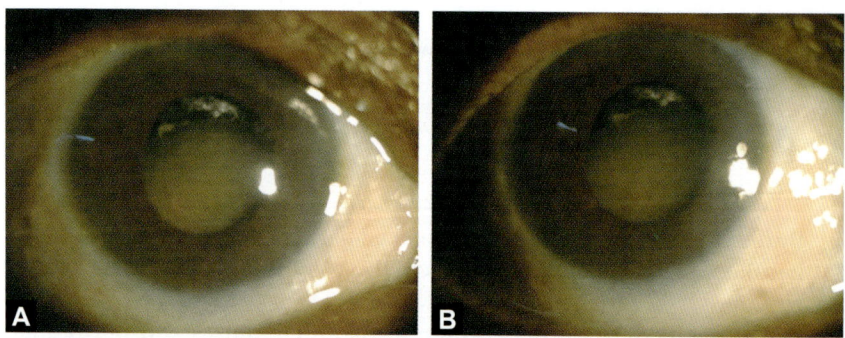

Figs 2A and B Gross view: (A) Straight position of eye, (B) Eye in upward gaze

Slit Lamp Examination

Gross View

1. Hypermature cataract.
2. Inferior subluxation.
3. Calcified capsular bag.

HYPERMATURE HARD CATARACT WITH INFERIOR SUBLUXATION (FIGS 3A AND B)

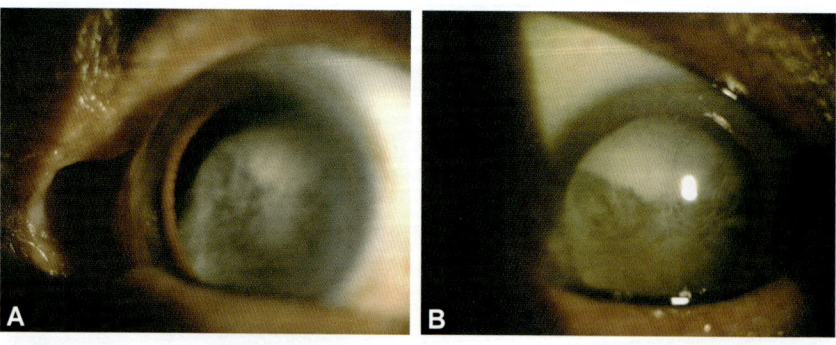

Figs 3A and B (A) Subluxation noticed in medial gaze of eye position, (B) Subluxation is not noticed in straight gaze of eye position

Slit Lamp Examination

Gross View

1. Hypermature hard cataract.
2. Wrinkling is seen on anterior capsule.

HYPERMATURE INTUMESCENT CATARACT (FIGS 4A AND B)

Slit Lamp Examination

Gross View

1. Hypermature milky cataract.
2. Zonular weakness is seen superiorly.

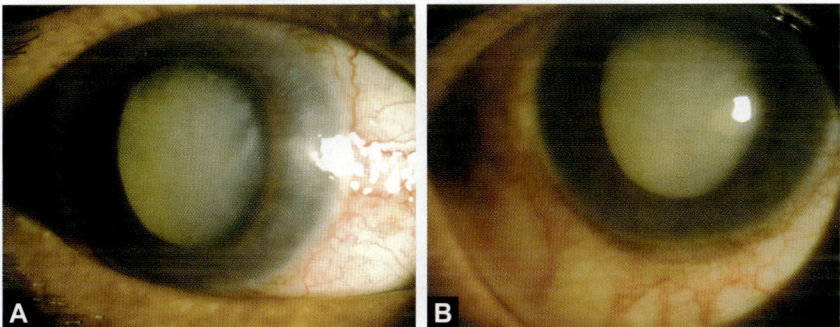

Figs 4A and B Gross view

HYPERMATURE HARD CATARACT (FIG. 5)

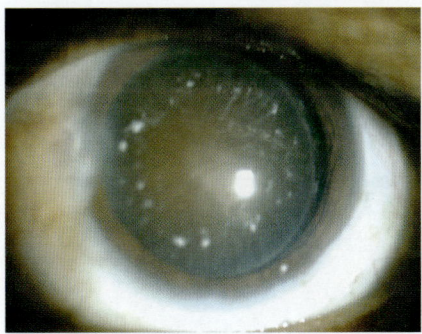

Fig. 5 Gross view

Slit Lamp Examination

Gross View

1. Hard cataract with more than 180 degrees subluxation
2. Calcified plaque seen on anterior capsule.

HYPERMATURE CATARACT WITH INFERIOR SUBLUXATION (FIG. 6)

Slit Lamp Examination

Gross View

1. Hypermature cataract.
2. Inferior subluxation.

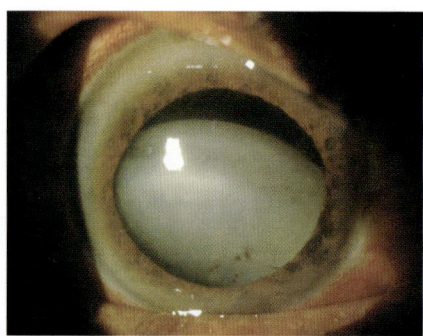

Fig. 6 Gross view

Advice (Figs 1 to 6)

1. Intracapsular cataract extraction (ICCE) with secondary IOL implantation can be considered.
2. Vitrectomy is needed in many cases.

IMMATURE CATARACT WITH MINIMAL SUBLUXATION (FIG. 7)

Slit Lamp Examination

Gross View

1. Subluxation from 7 to 9 o'clock.
2. Centrally located cataract.

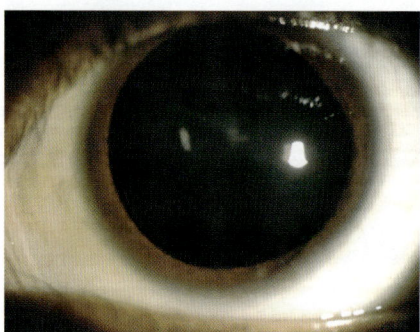

Fig. 7 Gross view

IMMATURE CATARACT WITH SUBLUXATION (FIGS 8A TO C)

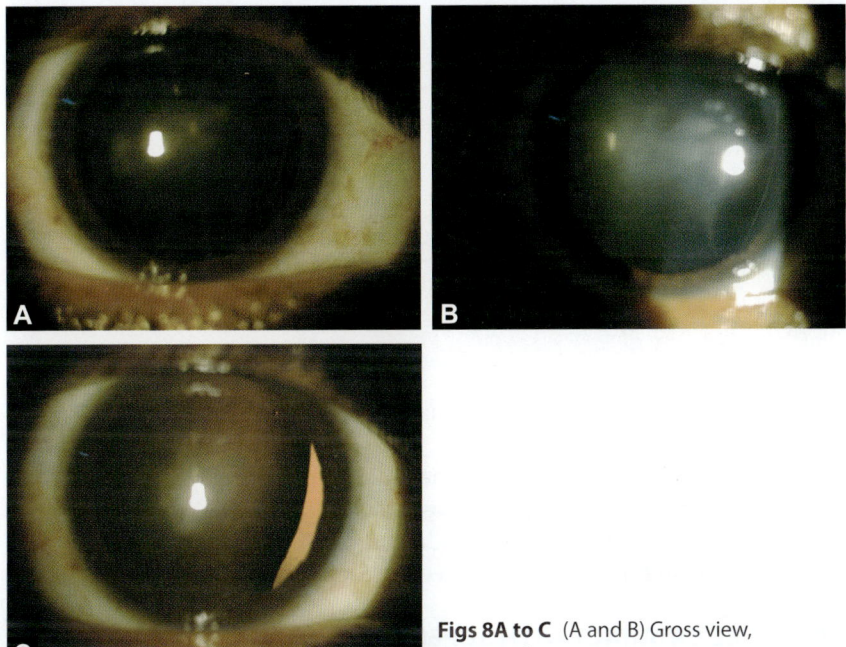

Figs 8A to C (A and B) Gross view, (C) Retroillumination

Slit Lamp Examination

Gross View

1. Subluxation is from 2 to 5 o'clock.
2. Confirmed in retroillumination.
3. Immature cataract.

POSTERIOR SUBCAPSULAR CATARACT WITH SUBLUXATION (FIGS 9A AND B)

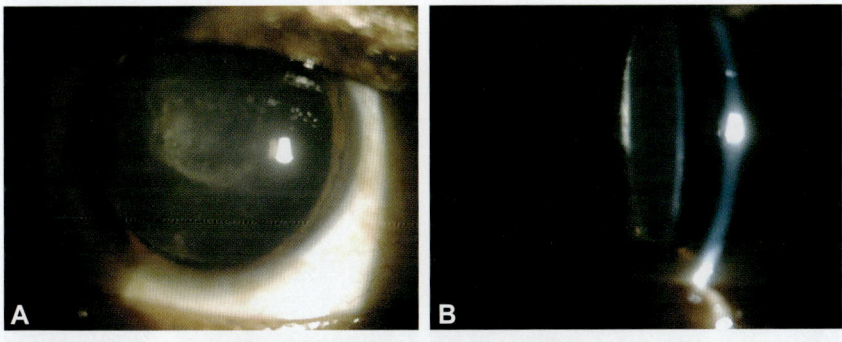

Figs 9A and B (A) Gross view, (B) Slit view

Slit Lamp Examination

Gross View

1. Posterior subcapsular cataract.
2. Subluxation is from 5 to 8 o'clock.

Slit View

1. Soft cataract.
2. Posterior subcapsular cataract (PSC) confirmed as an illuminated line.
3. No nucleus.

Advice (Figs 7 to 9)

1. Phaco surgery should be done.
2. Capsulorhexis should be of adequate size. Microcapsulorhexis forceps is helpful.
3. CTR to be inserted after capsulorhexis.
4. Rest of the nucleus management as in soft cataract.
5. Irrigation-aspiration is difficult due to CTR. Tangential movement of irrigation-aspiration cannula is needed for irrigation and aspiration.

IMMATURE CATARACT WITH SUPERIOR SUBLUXATION (FIGS 10A AND B)

Slit Lamp Examination

Gross View

1. Immature cataract.
2. Subluxated from 1 to 7 o'clock, i.e. more than 180 degrees.

Slit View

1. All layers of the lens are seen.
2. It is very soft cataract.

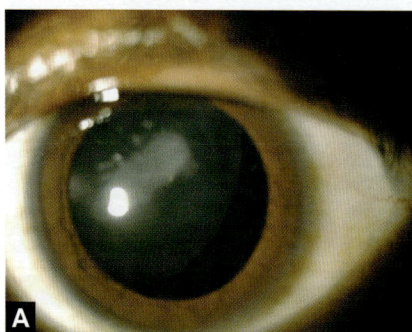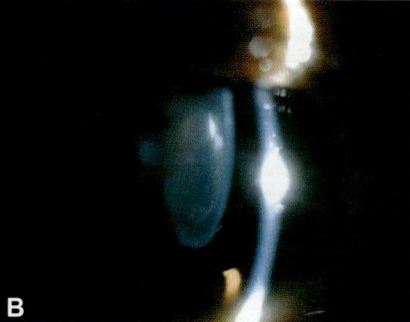

Figs 10A and B (A) Gross view, (B) Slit view

Advice

1. After capsulorhexis, which is the most challenging step, put the capsular hooks to support the capsule.
2. Nucleus management as in soft cataract.
3. Modified CTR or Ahmed segment should be used to support the bag at the subluxated site.

SUBLUXATED LENS AND CATARACT WITH MARFAN SYNDROME (FIGS 11A TO C)

Slit Lamp View

Gross View

1. Subluxation of lens is seen in superotemporal and superonasal position.
2. Well demarcated lens edge seen in retroillumination.

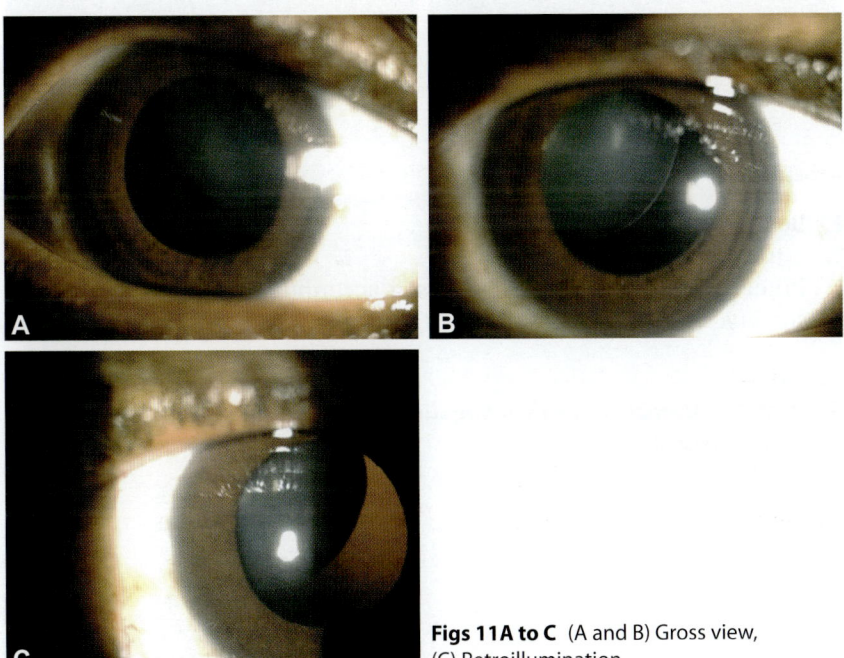

Figs 11A to C (A and B) Gross view, (C) Retroillumination

Advice

1. Lensectomy only.
2. Lensectomy with IOL implantation.
3. Secondary IOL after some period.
4. In all situations vitrectomy is needed.

MICROSPHEROPHAKIA (FIGS 12A AND B)

Slit Lamp Examination

Gross View

1. In undilated pupil surgeon has noticed subluxation.
2. Small spherical lens, which is dislocated anteriorly on dilatation.

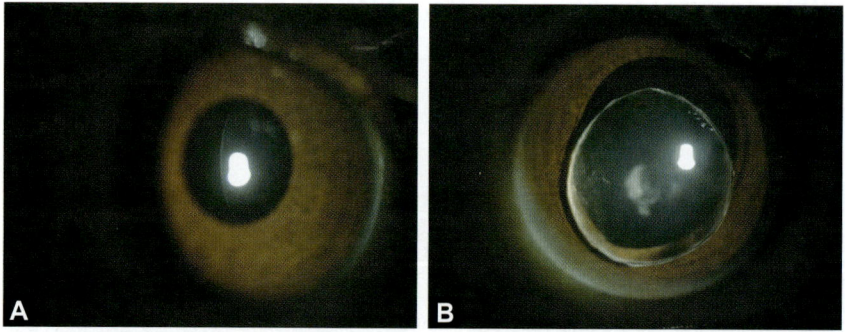

Figs 12A and B Gross view: (A) Undilated pupil, (B) After dilatation of pupil

Advice

1. Removal of the lens.
2. Vitrectomy is needed.
3. Primary or secondary IOL is advised according to the situation during surgery.

KEY NOTE

Subluxated cataract is a challenging situation for every surgeon. Management varies from case-to-case.

Section 3

Cataract with Associated Conditions and Factors

- Cataract with Pseudoexfoliation
- Cataract with Shallow Anterior Chamber
- Cataract with Small Pupil
- Cataract with Suspicious Weak Zonules
- Cataract with Corneal Opacity and Hazy Cornea
- Cataract with Different Shapes of Pupil
- Cataract with Hyperopia
- Cataract with Myopia
- Cataract with Embedded Foreign Body in the Lens
- Cataract with Floppy Iris Syndrome
- Cataract with Glaucoma
- Cataract with Iris Coloboma
- Cataract with Micro-ophthalmos
- Cataract with Vitreous Opacities
- Cataract with Pterygium
- Cataract with Mooren's Ulcer
- Cataract in Post-radial Keratotomy Case
- Cataract in Post-penetrating Keratoplasty Case
- Cataract in Post-trabeculectomy Cases
- Cataract in Young Age
- Cataract in Old Age
- Cataract with Uneven Anterior Chamber
- Cataract with Wrinkling of Face

Chapter 20

Cataract with Pseudoexfoliation

INTRODUCTION

1. Cataract is associated with pseudoexfoliation (PXE) in many cases.
2. One may miss this finding on torch light examination, but Slitlamp examination is important to find out signs of PXE.
3. On examination pseudoexfoliation material may be seen on corneal endothelium, at pupillary border and anterior lens capsule. These cases are quite often associated with glaucoma so detailed examination is necessary.
4. These cataract cases are not straight forward cases. Difficulties in these cases are due to hazy cornea, shallow anterior chamber, small pupil and variable density of the nucleus.
5. *Most crucial factor is suspicious zonular weakness which is most challenging factor. Other eye examination in these particular cases is very important.*

Management

Stop and chop technique of Phaco surgery is preferred.

1. Limbal incision is preferred so that conversion to SICS/ECCE is easy.
2. Capsulorhexis should be done within pseudoexfoliated material.
3. Minimal or no hydroprocedure
4. Trench should be done with adequate or more energy to avoid pressure on zonules.
5. Unnecessary rotation should be avoided.
6. Hold and lift of half piece of the nucleus should be done slowly.
7. Removal of pieces is as usual.
8. Irrigation-aspiration is difficult as there is suspicious zonular weakness.
9. Foldable intraocular lens (IOL) implantation should be done cautiously.

DIFFERENT VARIETY OF PSEUDOEXFOLIATION (FIGS 1A TO F)

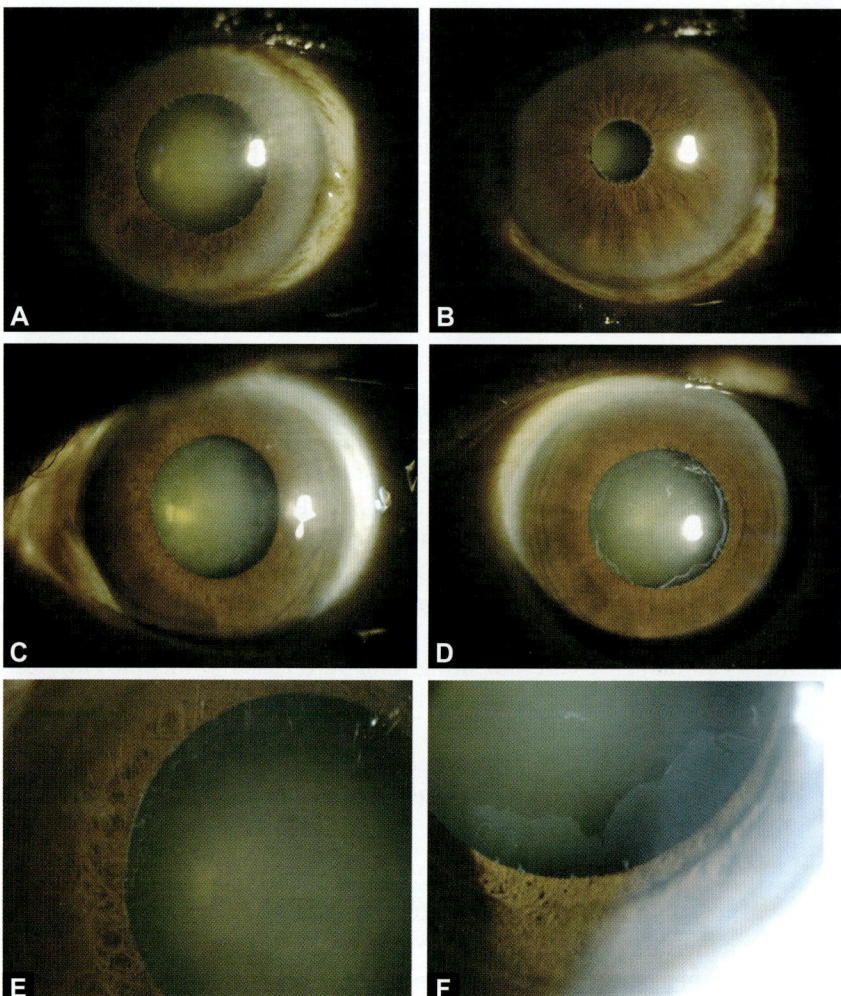

Figs 1A to F (A to D) Gross view, (E and F) Magnified view

PSEUDOEXFOLIATION WITH ADEQUATE SIZE OF NUCLEUS (FIGS 2A AND B)

Slit Lamp Examination

Gross View

1. PXE on anterior surface of the lens
2. Adequate size nucleus.

Chapter 20: Cataract with Pseudoexfoliation

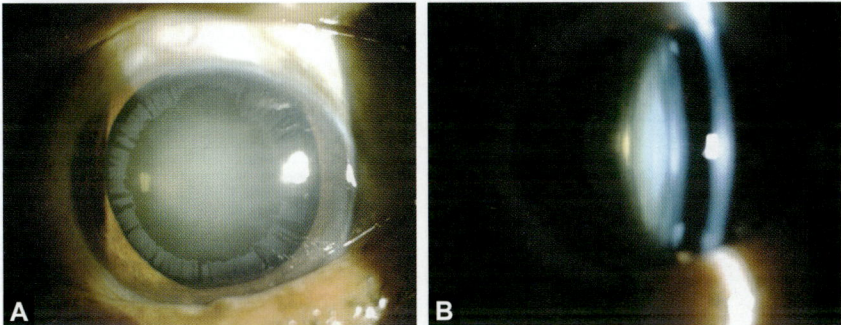

Figs 2A and B (A) Gross view, (B) Slit view

Slit View

1. All layers of the lens are seen
2. Grade 2, adequate size nucleus.

Advice

Phaco surgery is easy.

IMMATURE CATARACT WITH PXE (FIGS 3A AND B)

Slit Lamp Examination

Gross View

1. Pseudoexfoliation on anterior capsule 360 degrees
2. Mid-dilated pupil
3. Immature cataract.

Slit View

1. All layers of the lens are seen
2. Grade 2 dense, adequate size nucleus.

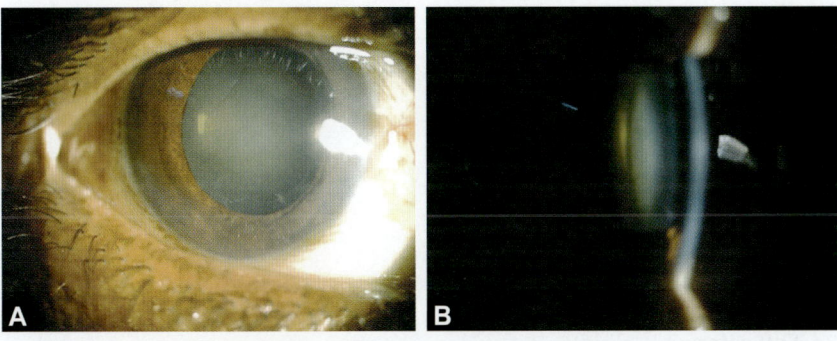

Figs 3A and B (A) Gross view, (B) Slit view

Advice

Phaco surgery is easy.

PSEUDOEXFOLIATION CATARACT WITH SMALL PUPIL (FIGS 4A AND B)

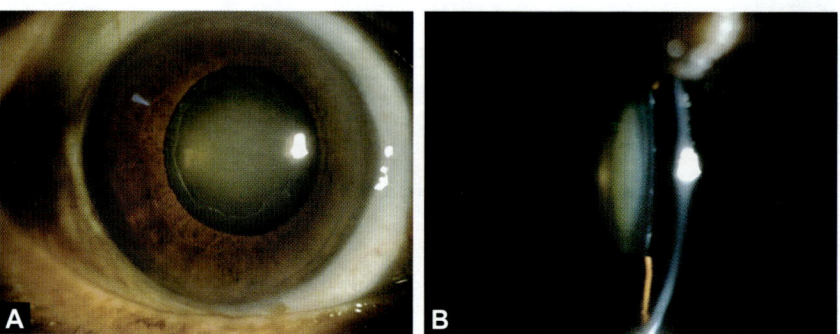

Figs 4A and B (A) Gross view, (B) Slit view

Slit Lamp Examination

Gross View

1. PXE on anterior capsule 360 degrees and pupillary border
2. Mid-dilated pupil.

Slit View

1. All layers of the lens are seen
2. Grade 2 dense, adequate size nucleus with PSC.

Advice

Phaco surgery is easy.

PSEUDOEXFOLIATION CATARACT WITH SMALL SIZE NUCLEUS (FIGS 5A TO C)

Slit Lamp Examination

Gross View

1. PXE on anterior capsule.
2. Pupil is dilated.
3. Immature cataract.

Slit View

1. All layers of the lens are seen.
2. Soft cataract.
3. Small size nucleus.

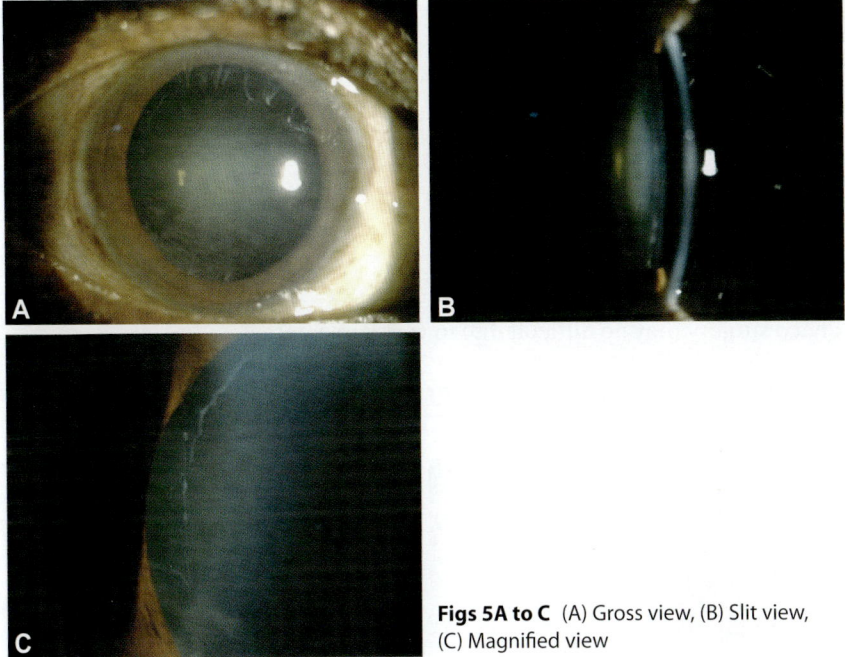

Figs 5A to C (A) Gross view, (B) Slit view, (C) Magnified view

Advice

Phaco surgery is easy.

PSEUDOEXFOLIATION WITH SOFT CATARACT (FIGS 6A AND B)

Slit Lamp Examination

Gross View

1. Soft cataract
2. Semidilated pupil

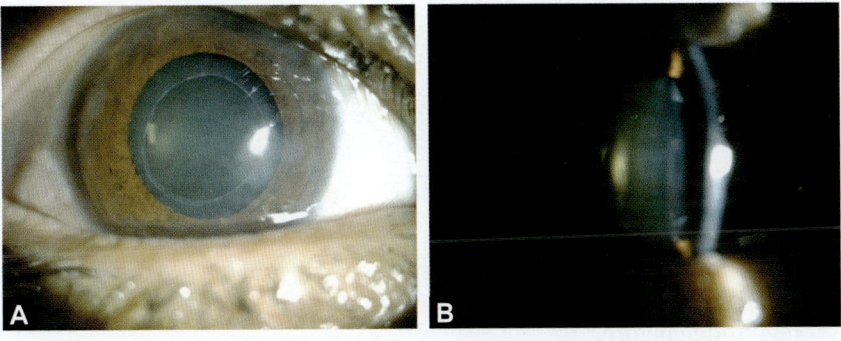

Figs 6A and B (A) Gross view, (B) Slit view

3. 360 degrees uniform PXE material on anterior capsule which mimics capsulorhexis
4. PXE is seen on pupillary border also.

Slit View

1. Soft cataract is confirmed
2. Grade 1 nucleus.

Advice

Phaco surgery may be difficult due to very soft cataract.

PSEUDOEXFOLIATION WITH HARD CATARACT (FIGS 7A AND B)

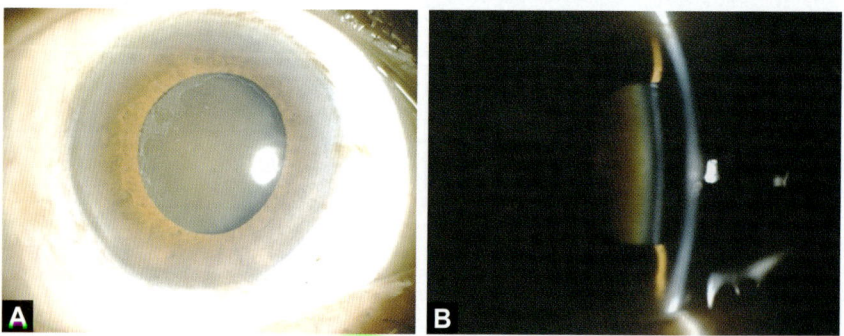

Figs 7A and B (A) Gross view, (B) Slit view

Slit Lamp Examination

Gross View

1. Hard cataract
2. Semidilated pupil.

Slit View

1. All layers of the lens are seen
2. Grade 5 to 6 dense nucleus, edges of nucleus hide behind pupillary area
3. AC seems to be shallow.

Advice

1. *Best option is to do SICS/ECCE.*
2. One can go ahead with the Phaco surgery by managing the pupil size with different ways and has to be confident to tackle hard cataract as mentioned before.

PSEUDOEXFOLIATION CATARACT WITH BULKY NUCLEUS (FIGS 8A AND B)

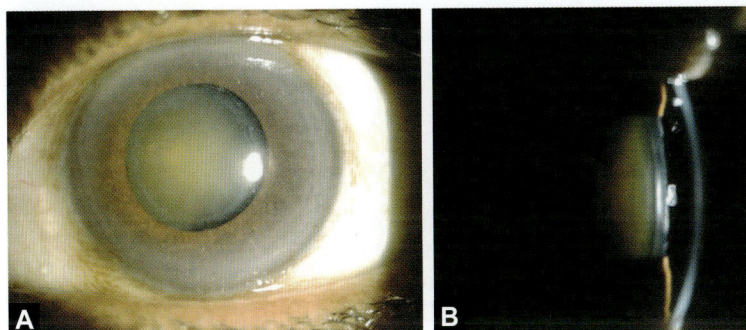

Figs 8A and B (A) Gross view, (B) Slit view

Slit Lamp Examination

Gross View

1. Hard cataract
2. Mid-dilated pupil
3. PXE material 360 degrees
4. Hazy cornea.

Slit View

1. All layers of the lens are seen
2. Grade 3 to 4 dense nucleus
3. Bulky but adequate size nucleus.

Advice

One can go ahead with Phaco surgery.

PSEUDOEXFOLIATION WITH MATURE CATARACT (FIGS 9A AND B)

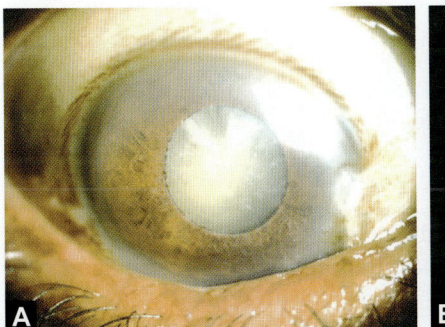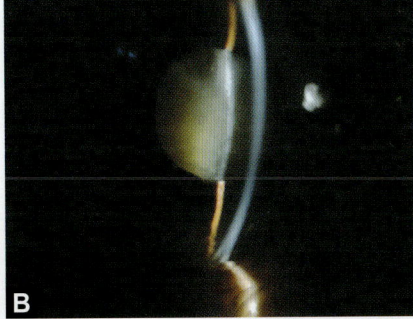

Figs 9A and B (A) Gross view, (B) Slit view

Slit Lamp Examination

Gross View

1. Mature cataract
2. Pupil is not fully dilated.

Slit View

All layers are not well defined.

Advice

1. Phaco surgery is always unpredictable
2. One can think of doing SICS/ECCE which may be safer option.

PSEUDOEXFOLIATION WITH CORTICAL CATARACT (FIGS 10A AND B)

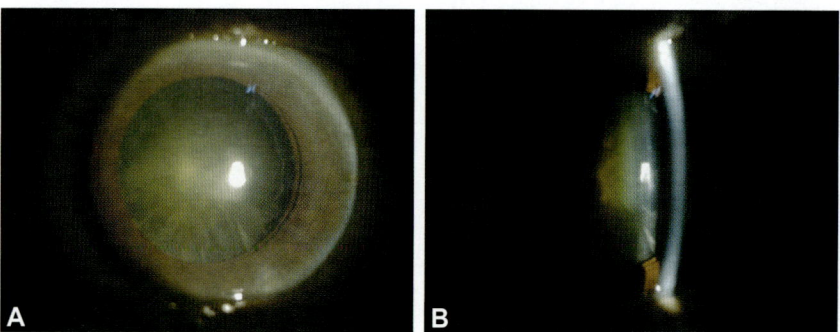

Figs 10A and B (A) Gross view, (B) Slit view

Slit Lamp Examination

Gross View

Pseudoexfoliation with cortical cataract.

Slit View

1. All layers of the lens are seen
2. Grade 2 nucleus with adequate size.

Advice

Phaco surgery can be done comfortably with precaution of hold and lift of half piece of nucleus and in irrigation-aspiration of epinucleus and cortex.

PSEUDOEXFOLIATION WITH BLACK CATARACT (FIGS 11A AND B)

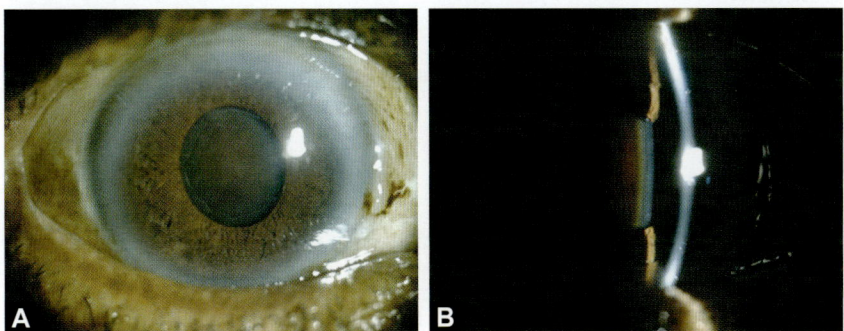

Figs 11A and B (A) Gross view, (B) Slit view

Slit Lamp Examination

Gross View

1. Very hard cataract
2. Pupil is not fully dilated.

Slit View

All layers of the lens are not seen.

Advice

Phaco surgery is difficult. SICS/ECCE is the surgery of choice.

PSEUDOEXFOLIATION WITH VERY HARD CATARACT (FIGS 12A AND B)

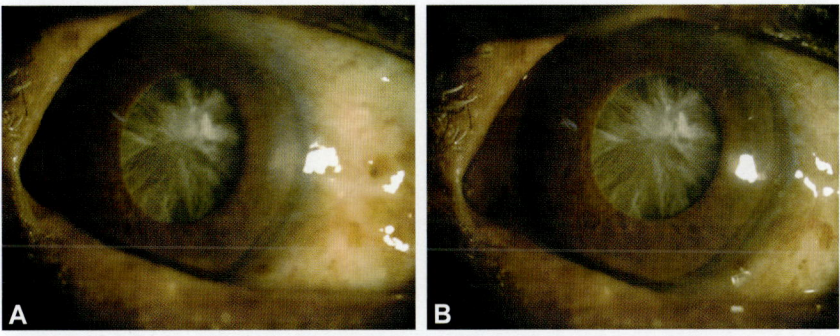

Figs 12A and B Gross view

Slit Lamp Examination

Gross View

1. Very hard cataract
2. Wrinkling of anterior capsule indicates zonular weakness
3. Pupil is not fully dilated.

Advice

SICS/ECCE is the surgery of choice.

KEY NOTE

Consideration of zonular weakness in pseudoexfoliation cataract is the most important factor.

Chapter 21

Cataract with Shallow Anterior Chamber

INTRODUCTION

1. This is most crucial situation for phaco surgery.
2. *Difficulty in surgery is due to less working space.*
3. Chances of haziness of the cornea and the posterior capsule rupture are quite common.
4. Shallow anterior chamber (AC) is usually associated with small or mid-dilated pupil.
5. Systematic approach is needed for these cases.
6. More incisions and more instrumentation inside the AC should be avoided.

CATARACT WITH SHALLOW ANTERIOR CHAMBER (FIGS 1A TO D)

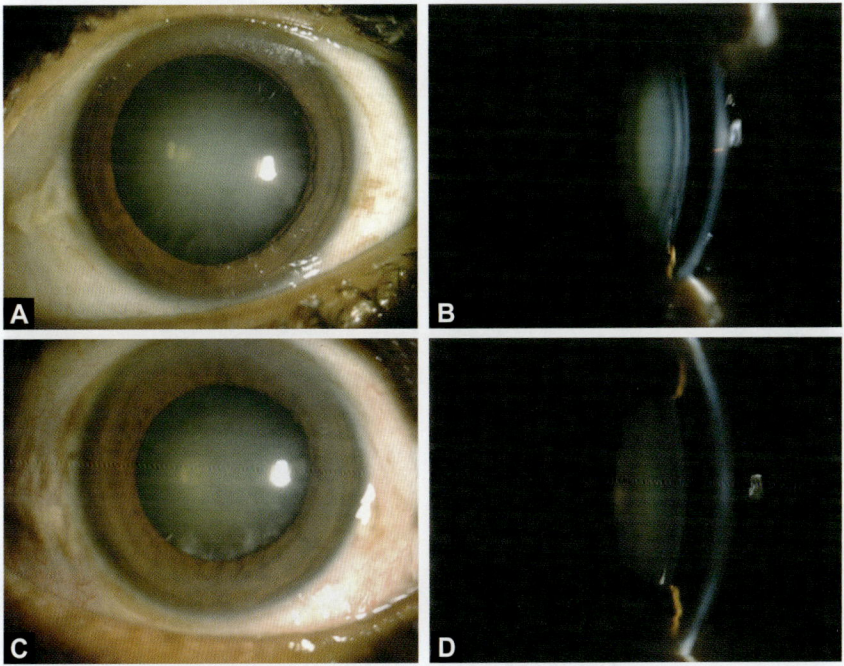

Figs 1A to D (A and C) Gross view, (B and D) Slit view

Slit Lamp Examination

Gross View

1. Clear cornea.
2. Mid-dilated pupil.
3. Adequate size and hardness of the nucleus.
4. Shallow AC.

Slit View

1. All layers of the lens are seen.
2. Convexity of the iris confirms shallow AC.
3. Grade 2 to 3 nucleus sclerosis with adequate size is confirmed.

Advice

1. Phaco surgery is easy.
2. Capsulorhexis should be small as there are chances of capsulorhexis run away.
3. Minimal or no hydro procedure.
4. Trench should be according to the size and density of nucleus.
5. In division, more attempts of division should be avoided as chances of collapse of anterior chamber is there.
6. Hold and lift should be restricted to the capsulorhexis border so that passing of chopper is easy.
7. Removal of small pieces should be done in the central safe zone mainly.
8. Irrigation-aspiration is difficult due to associated shallow bag.
9. IOL implantation should be done with caution as there is no much space.

DENSE NUCLEAR CATARACT WITH SHALLOW ANTERIOR CHAMBER (FIGS 2A AND B)

Slit Lamp Examination

Gross View

1. Mid-dilated pupil.
2. Dense nuclear cataract.

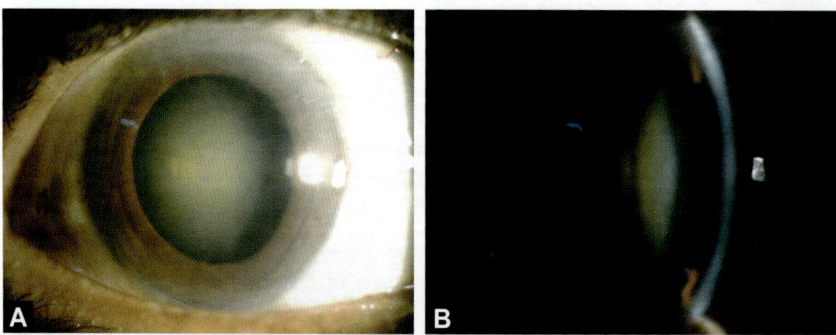

Figs 2A and B (A) Gross view, (B) Slit view

Slit View

1. All layers of the lens are seen.
2. Adequate hardness with adequate size nucleus.

Advice

Phaco surgery can be easily managed.

DENSE NUCLEAR CATARACT WITH HAZY CORNEA (FIGS 3A AND B)

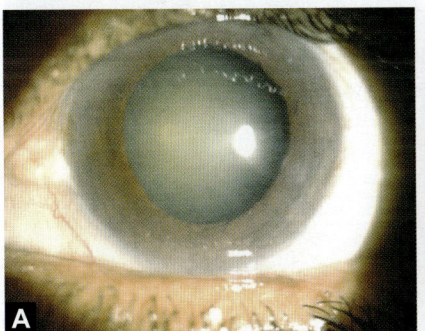 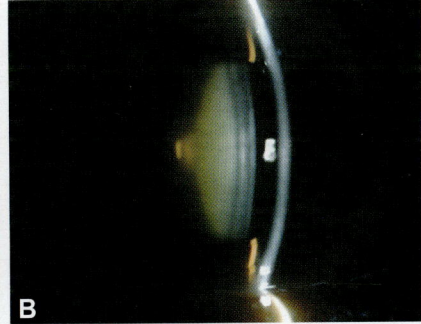

Figs 3A and B (A) Gross view, (B) Slit view

Slit Lamp Examination

Gross View

1. Mid-dilated pupil.
2. Hazy cornea.
3. Dense nuclear cataract.

Slit View

1. All layers of the lens are seen.
2. Big size dense nucleus is confirmed.

Advice

1. One can go ahead with Phaco surgery with all measures to be taken to avoid injury to the cornea.
2. Use of high molecular weight viscoelastic agents.
3. During removal of small pieces, bevel of the Phaco tip should be horizontal and directed away from cornea.
4. *Try to keep Phaco tip away from cornea throughout the nucleus management.*

MATURE CATARACT WITH SHALLOW ANTERIOR CHAMBER (FIGS 4A AND B)

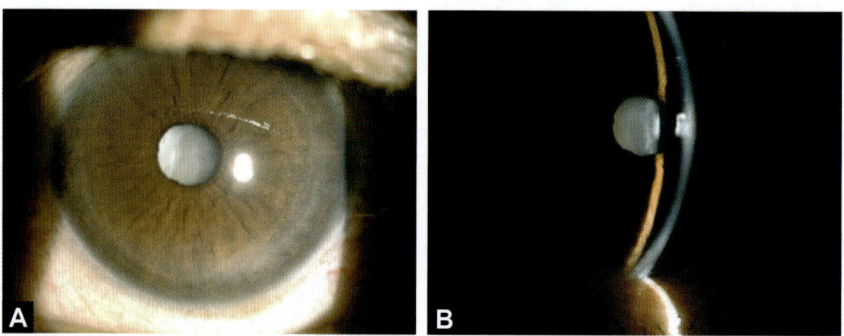

Figs 4A and B (A) Gross view, (B) Slit view

Slit Lamp Examination

Gross View

Mature cataract with shallow AC.

Slit View

1. Shallow AC is confirmed.
2. *Examination of the eye with undilated pupil will give correct idea about shallow AC, as many times after dilatation of the same eye, surgeon may feel AC is normal or deep which will give wrong information and may lead to difficulties in the surgery.*

Advice

Phaco surgery is not very easy.

PSEUDOEXFOLIATION CATARACT WITH SHALLOW ANTERIOR CHAMBER (FIGS 5A AND B)

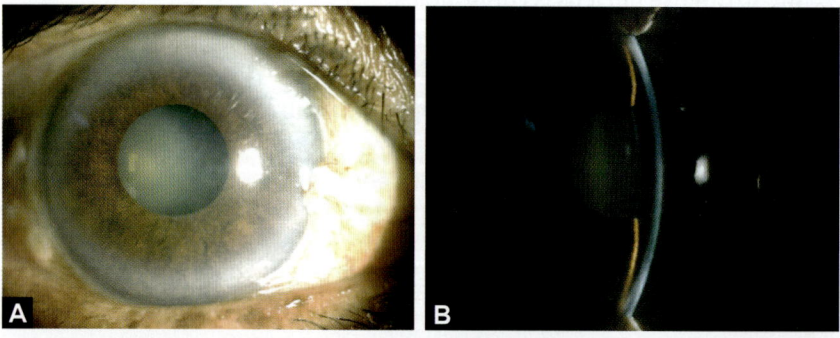

Figs 5A and B (A) Gross view, (B) Slit view

Slit Lamp Examination

Gross View

1. Shallow AC.
2. Pupil is not fully dilated.
3. Pseudoexfoliation cataract.

Slit View

Shallow AC is confirmed.

Pseudoexfoliation cataract is many times associated with shallow AC.

Advice

Phaco surgery has to be done with cautions.

SOFT CATARACT WITH SHALLOW ANTERIOR CHAMBER (FIGS 6A AND B)

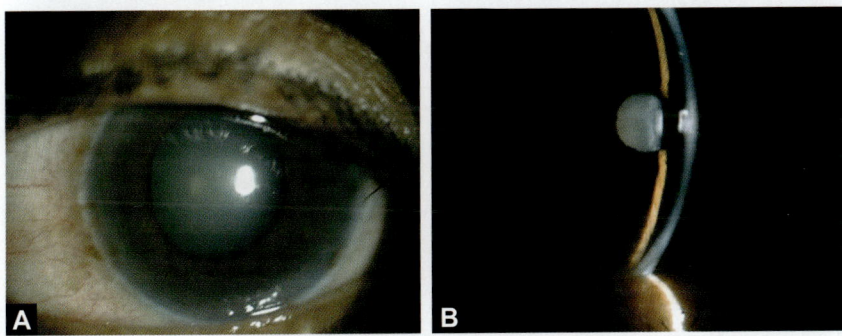

Figs 6A and B (A) Gross view, (B) Slit view

Slit Lamp Examination

Gross View

1. Shallow AC.
2. Mid-dilated pupil.
3. Soft cataract.

Slit View

Shallow AC is confirmed.

Advice

This is one of the deceiving situations for Phaco surgeons.

POSTOPERATIVE CASES IN SHALLOW ANTERIOR CHAMBER AND THE OTHER EYE (FIGS 7A TO D)

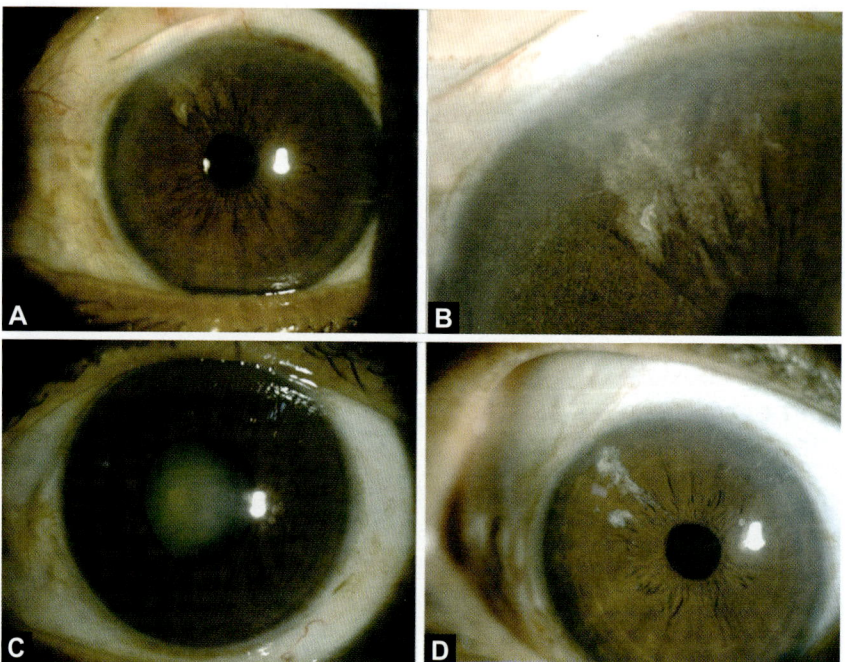

Figs 7A to D (A, C, D) Gross view, (B) Magnified view

Slit Lamp Examination

1. These atrophic patches of the iris at incision site in pseudophakic eye can give a clue of shallowness of AC.
2. Such type of findings in one eye will suggest anatomy of shallow AC in other eye with cataract.
3. These atrophic patches are due to rubbing of the iris during entry and exit of instruments during surgery and/or chances of iris prolapsed during surgery due to shallow AC.

KEY NOTE
Difficulty for Phaco surgery in shallow AC is due to less working space than normal.

Chapter 22

Cataract with Small Pupil

INTRODUCTION

1. This is a condition where the pupil remains small or mid dilated after instillation of dilating eye drops.
2. Small pupil cataract is associated with immature, mature, hard cataract, posterior synechiae and pseudoexfoliation. *Small pupil is usually associated with shallow anterior chamber.*
3. These cases need special management with respect to the pupil. Dilatation of pupil can be done by stretching of the iris, sometimes sphincterotomies, iris hooks, Malyugin ring and by some new devices.
4. Consideration of hardness and size of nucleus is important. In this variety of cases Phaco surgery can not be done in casual way.

IMMATURE CATARACT WITH SMALL PUPIL (FIGS 1A AND B)

Slit Lamp Examination

Gross View

Immature cataract is confirmed by iris shadow on the lens.

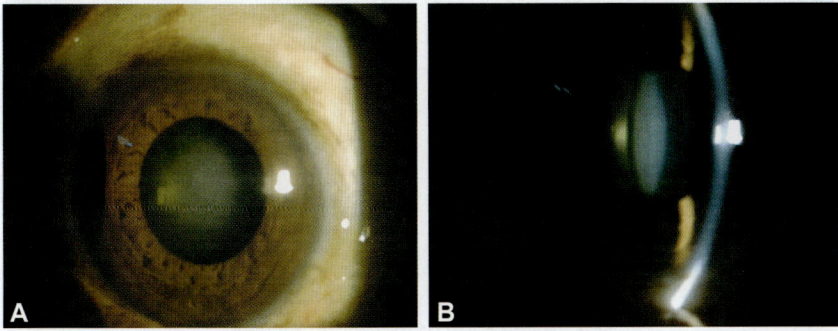

Figs 1A and B (A) Gross view, (B) Slit view

Slit View

1. All layers of the lens are seen.
2. Grade 2 nucleus with adequate size.

Advice

Phaco surgery can be easily done.
1. Capsulorhexis should be small.
2. Trench should be small in length.
3. Area of working is also small for further steps like hold and lift, and removal of small pieces, so chances of catching the pupillary border is more and parameters should be kept on the lower side.
4. Irrigation-aspiration is blind procedure here and should be done with cautions.
5. Intraocular lens (IOL) implantation is also difficult, Toric IOLs can be avoided as placement of lens is difficult in some cases.

NEARLY MATURE CATARACT WITH SMALL PUPIL (FIGS 2A AND B)

Slit Lamp Examination

Gross View

Nearly mature cataract.

Slit View

1. All layers of the lens are well defined.
2. Grade 3 with big size and bulky nucleus.

Advice

Phaco surgery can be done with all considerations of mature cataract.

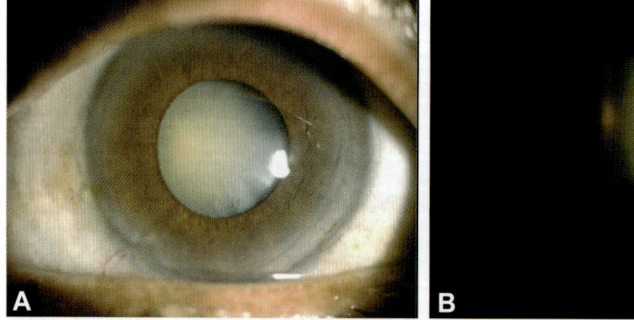

Figs 2A and B (A) Gross view, (B) Slit view

HARD CATARACT WITH SMALL PUPIL (FIGS 3A AND B)

Slit Lamp Examination

Gross View

1. Small pupil associated with hazy cornea.
2. Hard nucleus and diffuse cortical cataract.

Slit View

1. Hard and brown cataract with shadow of cortical cataract seen on the lens.
2. All layers of the lens are seen hazily.

Advice

1. Phaco surgery is difficult.
2. It can be avoided or can be done in cautious way.
3. More expertization is needed to tackle this situation.
4. *Difficulty is due to mismatch of dilatation of pupil related to hard and big size nucleus.*

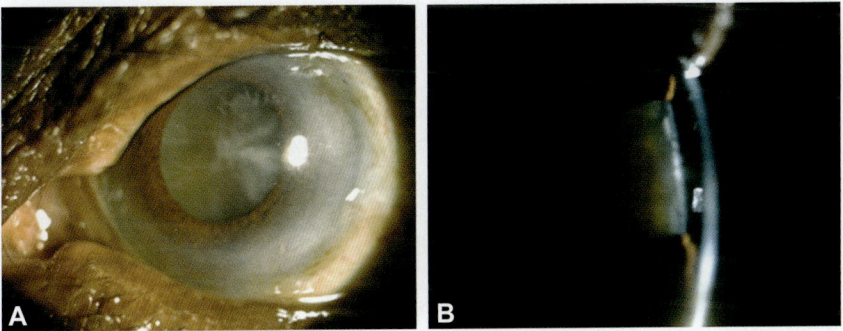

Figs 3A and B (A) Gross view, (B) Slit view

KEY NOTE

In examination, consideration of anatomy of the nucleus with respect to pupil size is very important. Management of small pupil is needed.

Chapter 23

Cataract with Suspicious Weak Zonules

INTRODUCTION

1. These cataract cases where one can suspect zonular weakness prior to surgery.
2. Some of the conditions like very old age, hard cataract, mature or hypermature cataract, pseudoexfoliation cataract, post-trabeculectomized eye, post-vitrectomized eye, myopia, cataract with wrinkling of skin of the face where one should suspect zonular weakness.
3. *This topic is important in the sense that in suspicious cases, one should be ready to tackle or to take all precautions to avoid further damage to capsular bag during surgery.*

Modifications in Phaco surgery is as follows:
1. Capsulorhexis should be small or adequate size.
2. No hydroprocedure or minimal hydroprocedure.
3. Trench with adequate or more energy.
4. Division with prechopper which gives equal pressure on two halves of nucleus.
5. Hold and lift of half part of nucleus should be done very slowly.
6. Removal of small pieces as a routine.
7. Irrigation-aspiration should be done cautiously.
8. Fill the bag with viscoelastics before Phaco probe or irrigation-aspiration cannula is taken out of anterior chamber.
9. Foldable intraocular lens (IOL) to be inserted without pressure on the bag.

CATARACT WITH WRINKLE ON ANTERIOR CAPSULE (FIGS 1A AND B)

Slit Lamp Examination

Gross View

1. Wrinkling on capsule is seen in cataract.
2. Other eye although normal one can suspect same zonular weakness which may be subclinical.

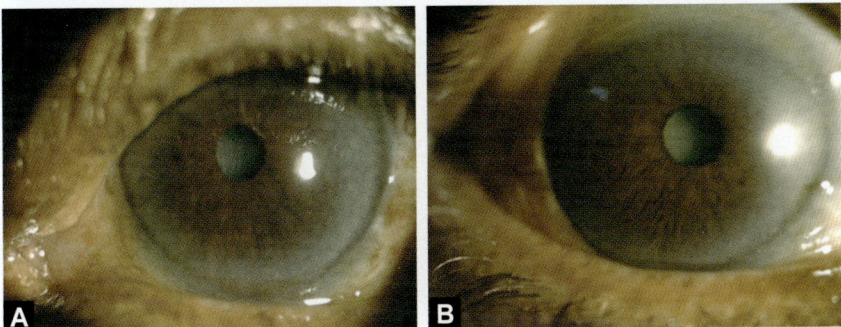

Figs 1A and B Gross view

CATARACT IN POST-TRABECULECTOMIZED EYE (FIG. 2)

Slit Lamp Examination

Gross View

Post-trabeculectomized eye with immature cataract where there is a possibility that zonules has been damaged during filtering surgery.

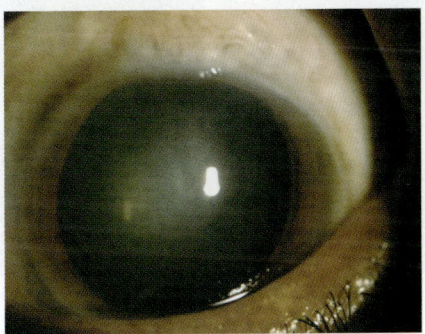

Fig. 2 Gross view

CATARACT WITH WEAK ZONE (FIG. 3)

Slit Lamp Examination

Gross View

Immature cataract with weak zone at 7 to 9 o' clock.

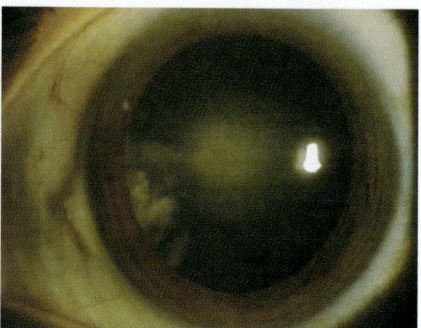

Fig. 3 Gross view

VERY HARD CATARACT (FIGS 4A AND B)

Slit Lamp Examination

Gross View and Slit View

Very hard cataract which means more degeneration.

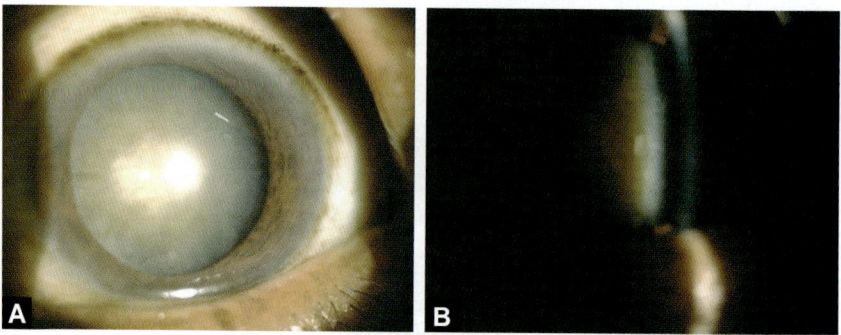

Figs 4A and B (A) Gross view, (B) Slit view

HYPERMATURE CATARACT WITH FIBROTIC ANTERIOR CAPSULE (FIG. 5)

Slit Lamp Examination

Gross View

Hypermature cataract with fibrotic anterior capsule.

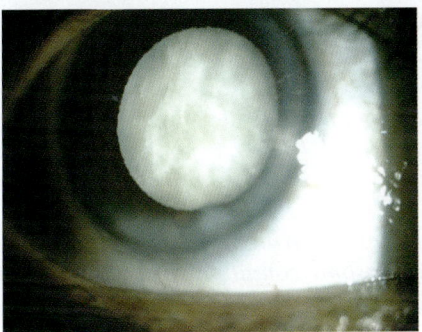

Fig. 5 Gross view

CATARACT WITH PSEUDOEXFOLIATION (FIG. 6)

Slit Lamp Examination

Gross View

1. Pseudoexfoliation cataract.
2. Pseudoexfoliated material seen at the pupillary border.

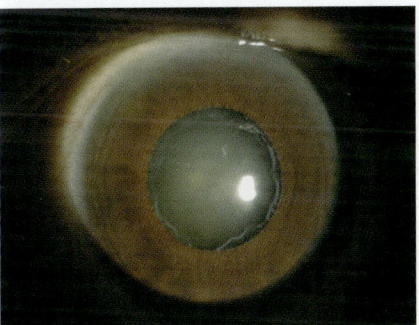

Fig. 6 Gross view

VERY OLD AGE CATARACT (FIGS 7A AND B)

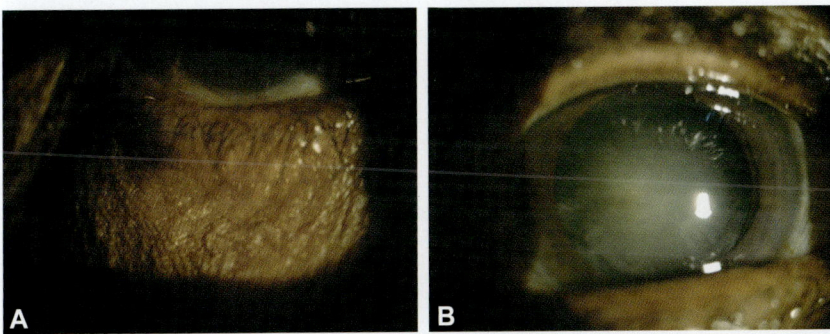

Figs 7A and B Gross view

Slit Lamp Examination

Gross View

Wrinkling on the face means more degeneration, so one can suspect zonular weakness in such cases.

KEY NOTE

One has to make the mind during cataract examination in routine practice to find out or correlate some conditions like old age, mature cataract, hard cataract, etc. with zonular weakness which is not obvious.

Chapter 24

Cataract with Corneal Opacity and Hazy Cornea

INTRODUCTION

1. Cataract with hazy cornea and corneal opacity are commonly seen complicated cases in practice.
2. Another factor is when surgeon noticed haziness in cornea, one should take in consideration the quality and quantity of endothelial cells. Specular microscopy is important in such situations.
3. Most important difficulty is visualization of steps of Phaco surgery. High molecular weight viscoelastic agents are important in this situation. Most of the time conversion from Phaco to small incision cataract surgery (SICS) or extracapsular cataract extraction (ECCE) is needed.

DENSE CATARACT WITH CENTRAL CORNEAL OPACITY (FIGS 1A AND B)

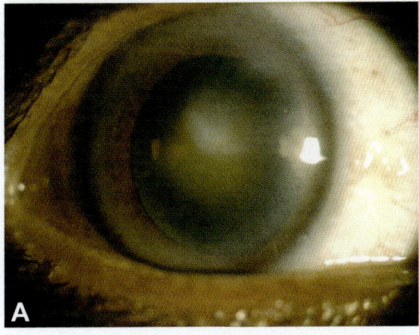
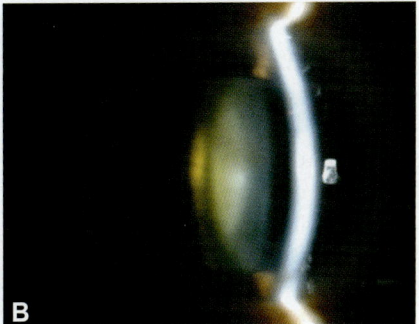

Figs 1A and B (A) Gross view, (B) Slit view

Slit Lamp Examination

Gross View

1. Central dense cataract.
2. Central corneal opacity.

3. Hazy cornea.
4. Pupil is not fully dilated.

Slit View

1. All layers of the lens are seen.
2. Grade 3 dense nucleus.
3. Adequate size of nucleus surrounded by sheet of epinucleus.
4. Posterior subcapsular cataract element is seen.

Advice

Phaco surgery can be performed as there is no major difficulty for visualization during surgery.

IMMATURE CATARACT WITH PERIPHERAL CORNEAL OPACITIES (FIGS 2A AND B)

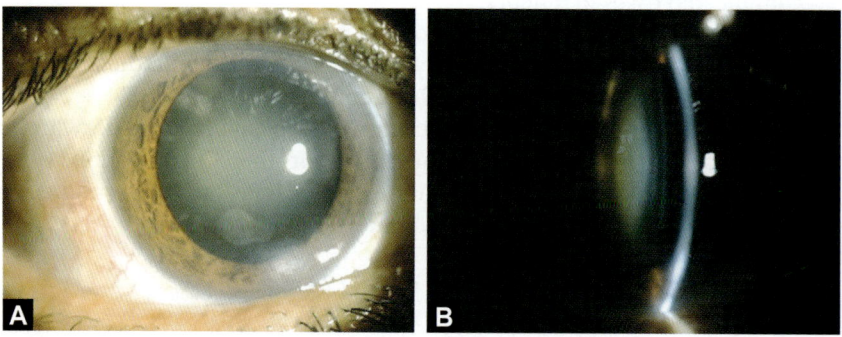

Figs 2A and B (A) Gross view, (B) Slit view

Slit Lamp Examination

Gross View

1. Immature cataract.
2. Peripheral corneal opacities.
3. Fully dilated pupil.

Slit View

1. All layers of the lens are seen.
2. Grade 2 dense nucleus.
3. Adequate size of the nucleus.
4. Corneal opacity marks are well noticed with slit beam on corneal layer.

Advice

Phaco surgery is easy.

DENSE CATARACT WITH HAZY CORNEA (FIGS 3A AND B)

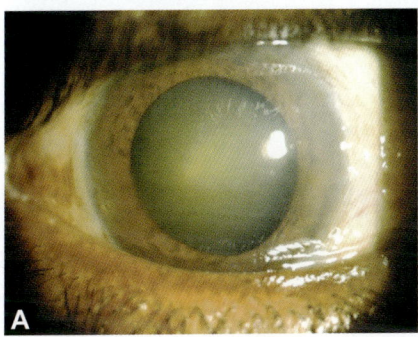 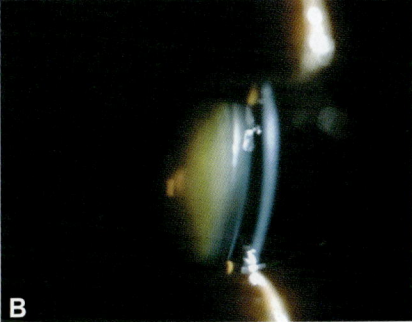

Figs 3A and B (A) Gross view, (B) Slit view

Slit Lamp Examination

Gross View

1. Dense cataract.
2. Hazy cornea.

Slit View

1. All layers of the lens are seen.
2. Grade 3 dense nucleus.
3. Adequate or slightly big size nucleus.

Advice

1. Phaco surgery can be performed.
2. High molecular weight viscoelastic solutions are needed.
3. Phaco probe and irrigation-aspiration cannula should be away from cornea.

DENSE CATARACT WITH INFERIOR CORNEAL OPACITY (FIGS 4A AND B)

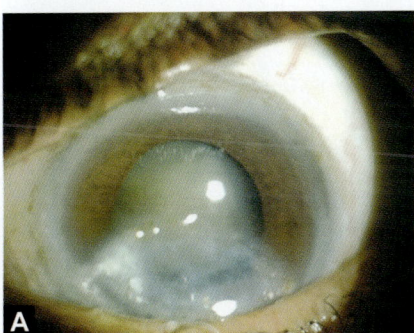 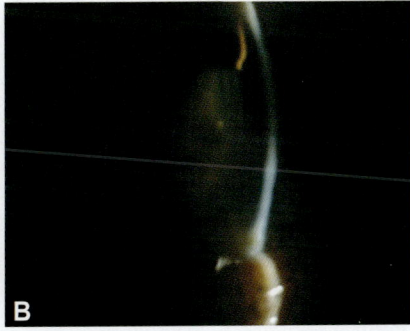

Figs 4A and B (A) Gross view, (B) Slit view

Slit Lamp Examination

Gross View

1. Dense cataract.
2. Inferior corneal opacity.
3. Pupil is not fully dilated.

Slit View

All layers of the lens are seen but hazily.

Advice

1. Phaco surgery can be done but with difficulty.
2. Conversion to SICS or ECCE is a simple option.

HARD CATARACT WITH CORNEAL OPACITY (FIGS 5A AND B)

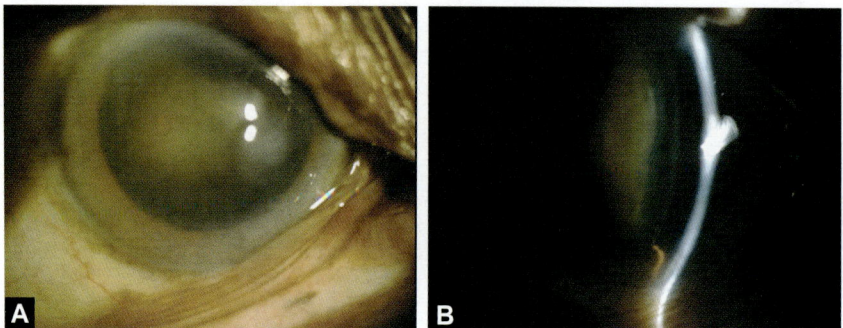

Figs 5A and B (A) Gross view, (B) Slit view

Slit Lamp Examination

Gross View

1. Very hard cataract.
2. Corneal opacity with hazy cornea.
3. Dilated pupil.

Slit View

1. All layers of the lens are seen hazily.
2. Wavy slit image on the lens confirms irregular cornea.
3. Grade 4 to 5 dense nucleus.
4. Big but still adequate size of nucleus.

Advice

1. Phaco surgery can be performed with consideration as a hard cataract management.
2. High molecular weight viscoelastic solutions are needed.
3. Conversion to SICS or ECCE is the safest way of thinking.

Followings are the situations of cataract with corneal opacity where one should think SICS or ECCE instead of Phaco surgery **(Figs 6 and 7)**.

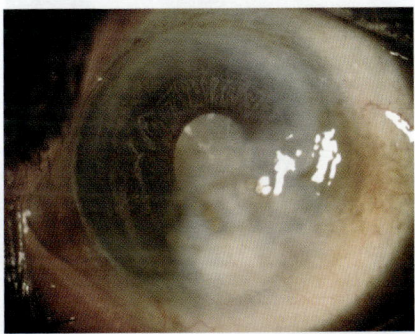

Fig. 6A Gross view: A hypermature cataract with inferior corneal opacity

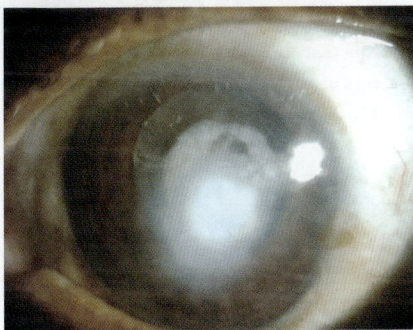

Fig. 6B Gross view: Hypermature cataract with central corneal opacity

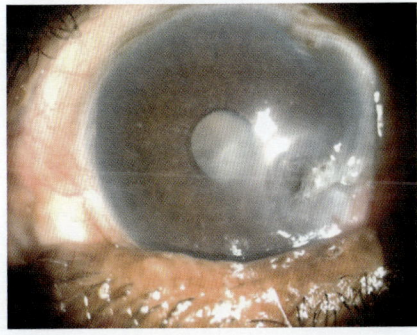

Fig. 6C Gross view: Mature cataract with corneal opacity at 4 to 5 o'clock position

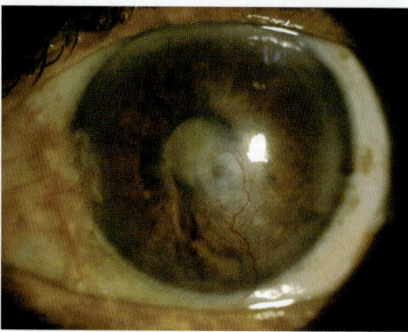

Fig. 6D Gross view: Hard and mature cataract with corneal opacity with vascularization

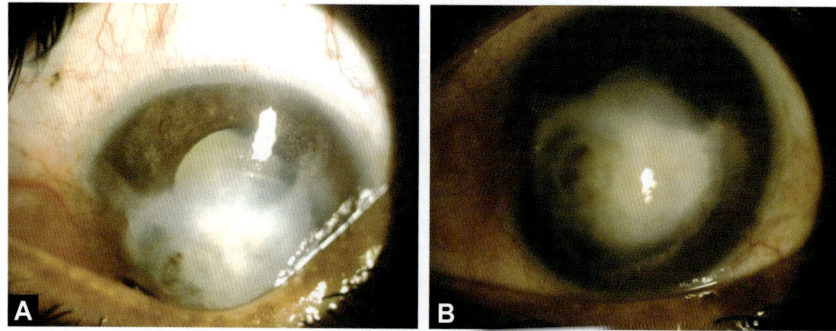

Figs 7A and B Gross view: Mature cataract with central corneal opacity (A) Downward gaze, (B) Straight gaze

Advice

1. Consideration of anterior chamber depth in every case is important for cataract management.
2. Although Phaco surgery can be performed in some cases, conversion to SICS or ECCE should is safe.

KEY NOTE
Most important difficulty for cataract surgery in these situations is visualization of the steps.

Chapter 25

Cataract with Different Shapes of Pupil

INTRODUCTION

1. Cataract with different shapes of the pupil is not uncommon finding seen in practice.
2. Pupil which is not central, round as a regular pupil is labeled as a different shape of pupil.
3. Pupil may be updrawn, temporally or nasally shifted or sometimes drawn downward.
4. Causes are congenital, injury, uveitis, post-glaucomatous surgical eyes, surgical iridectomy done in childhood for corneal opacity cases.
5. Cataract management depends on shape, size of pupil and types of cataract.

DIFFERENT PUPIL WITH NEARLY MATURE CATARACT (FIGS 1A TO C)

Slit Lamp Examination

Gross View

1. This is different pupil which is stretched towards 7 to 8 o' clock.
2. Nearly mature cataract.
3. After dilatation festoon shaped pupil.

Slit View

1. All layers of the lens are seen.
2. Grade 2 to 3 dense nucleus.
3. Adequate size of nucleus.

Advice

1. Phaco surgery can be possible with management of pupil.
2. Sometimes sphincterotomies are also needed to open central visual axis.

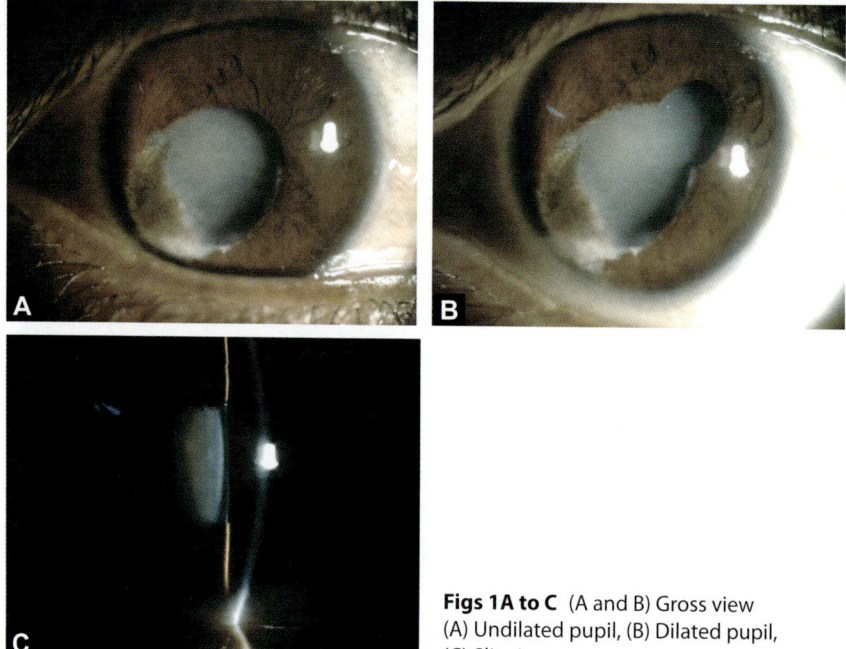

Figs 1A to C (A and B) Gross view (A) Undilated pupil, (B) Dilated pupil, (C) Slit view

KEY NOTE

This unusual condition can be easily managed by slit lamp examination of cataract in predilated and postdilated stage of pupil and management concerned with pupil.

Chapter 26

Cataract with Hyperopia

INTRODUCTION

1. This is a very common association seen in practice.
2. *This situation is also associated with small eyeball and shallow anterior chamber.*
3. All the special precautions of Phaco surgery are related to shallow anterior chamber and shallow capsular bag.

IMMATURE CATARACT (FIGS 1A TO D)

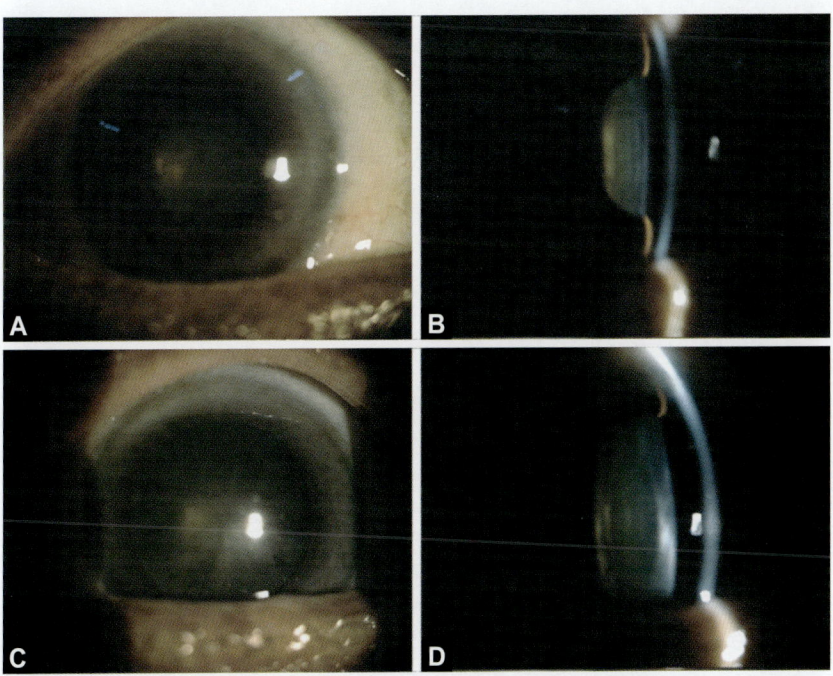

Figs 1A to D (A and C) Gross view, (B and D) Slit view

Slit Lamp Examination

Gross View

Diffuse and soft cataract.

Slit View

1. All layers of the lens are seen.
2. Shallow anterior chamber is confirmed.
3. Grade 1 to 2 dense nucleus.
4. Posterior subcapsular element is also seen.

Advice

1. *Phaco surgery is easy but the main difficulty is the less working space.*
2. Consideration of variety of foldable intraocular lenes is related to the space of the capsular bag.
3. Hydrophobic lenses are preferred.
4. Hydrophilic lenses should be avoided in shallow bag as these are bulky lenses than hydrophobic lenses.

KEY NOTE

Most important point of consideration in such cases is the shallow anterior chamber and management of cataract is mainly related to this factor.

Chapter 27

Cataract with Myopia

INTRODUCTION

1. This is one of the challenging situations for any Phaco surgeon.
2. This is usually soft cataract or many times clear lens extraction may be needed. *Other factors like hypotony, deep anterior chamber, deep capsular bag has to be considered throughout the procedure.*
3. Incision is difficult.
4. Capsulorhexis is easy.
5. After hydro procedure trench is as usual.
6. Division may be difficult.
7. Hold and lift and removal of pieces are easy as there is more space.
8. Sudden hypotony should be avoided by putting visco through the side port during removing of Phaco probe.
9. Irrigation-aspiration is difficult due to hypotony.
10. Foldable intraocular lens (IOL) implantation is also done with cautions, chances of tumbling of foldable IOL is more due to more space, i.e. deep anterior chamber and deep capsular bag.

IMMATURE CATARACT IN YOUNG PATIENT (FIGS 1A TO C)

Slit Lamp Examination

Gross View

1. Immature cataract.
2. Red glow is seen.

Slit View

1. All layers of the lens are seen.
2. Diffuse cortical cataract with no nucleus.
3. Soft variety of cataract.

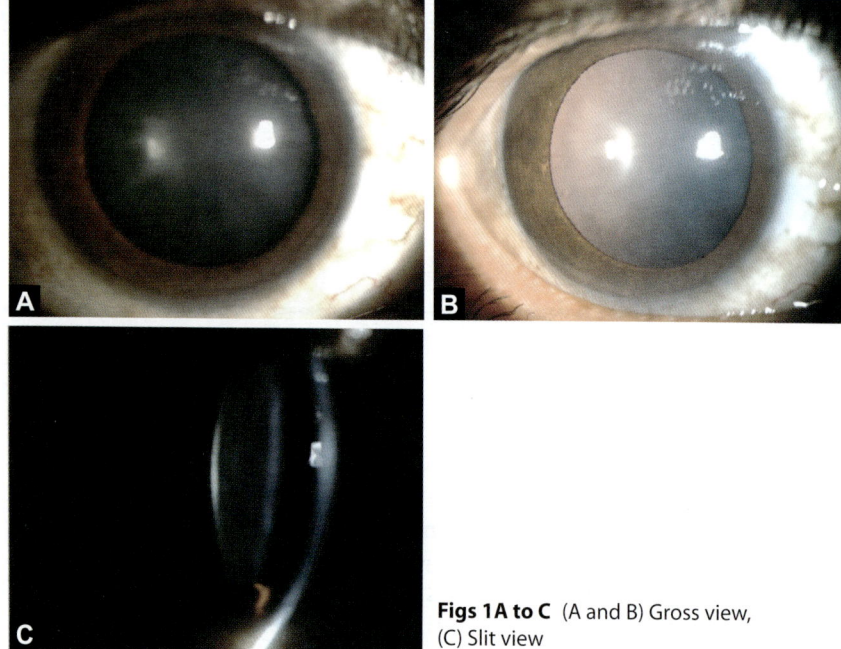

Figs 1A to C (A and B) Gross view, (C) Slit view

Advice

1. These cases should not be taken very casually.
2. Soft cataract management is needed.

KEY NOTE

Frequent change of the focus of the microscope is needed throughout the procedure due to deep AC or hypotony.

Chapter 28

Cataract with Embedded Foreign Body in the Lens

INTRODUCTION

1. Cataract with embedded foreign body is found secondary to injury with sharp object.
2. Foreign body will go inside and stay within the lens.
3. In this situation no specific different treatment is needed for this intraocular foreign body, removal of cataract will serve the purpose.

CATARACT WITH EMBEDDED FOREIGN BODY (FIGS 1A TO C)

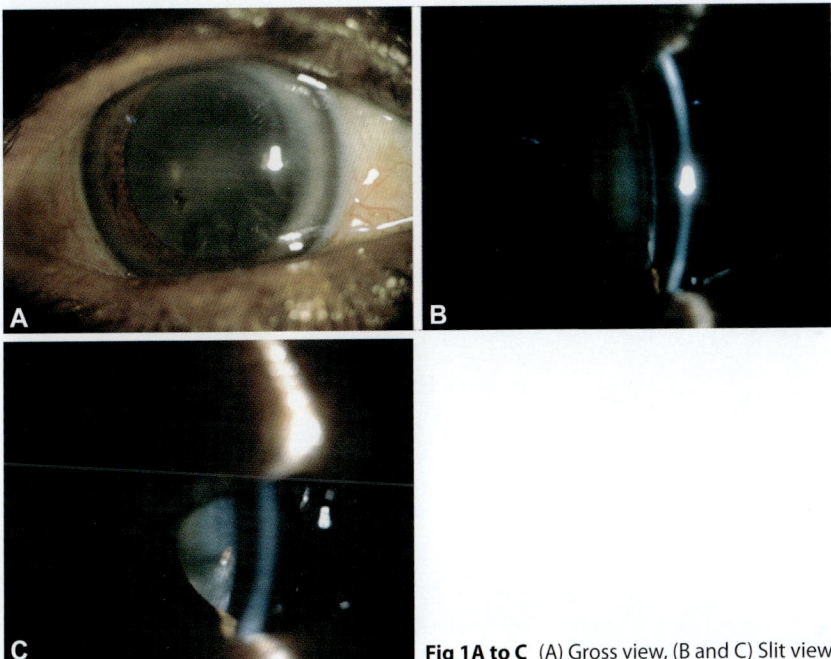

Fig 1A to C (A) Gross view, (B and C) Slit view

Slit Lamp Examination

Gross View

Immature cataract with localized brownish iron foreign body.

Slit View

1. Foreign body is confirmed.
2. All layers of the nucleus are seen which is grade 1 to 2 dense with adequate size.

Advice

1. Can be managed as a routine Phaco surgery.
2. Foreign body can get stuck in Phaco tip or irrigation/aspiration canula or tubings.

KEY NOTE

This is not a commonly seen condition which is managed by simple cataract extraction.

Chapter 29

Cataract with Floppy Iris Syndrome

INTRODUCTION
1. Iris is fragile in these situations.
2. In Phaco surgery one should take all the precautions to avoid injury to the iris which is already compromised.
3. Even with irrigating fluid also, iris can become more floppy and loose during surgery so that overall surgical time should be reduced to avoid more damage to the iris.

HARD CATARACT WITH FLOPPY IRIS (FIGS 1A TO C)

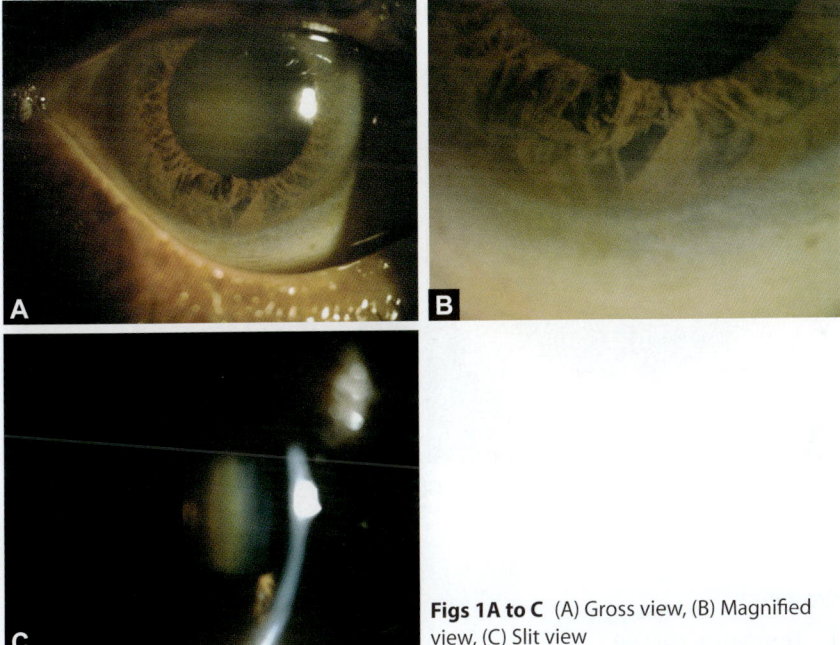

Figs 1A to C (A) Gross view, (B) Magnified view, (C) Slit view

Slit Lamp Examination

Gross View

1. Hard cataract
2. Floppy iris at 6 and 7 o'clock position
3. Pupil is not fully dilated.

Slit View

1. All layers of the lens are seen
2. Grade 3 to 4 dense nucleus
3. Size of the nucleus is more with respect to pupillary size
4. PSC element is also seen.

Advice

1. Phaco surgery can be done
2. Capsulorhexis should be small
3. Trench is according to size and density of nucleus. Direction should be away from abnormal iris
4. In division, due to dense PSC (sticky cataract) division may be difficult
5. During hold and lift, and removal of small pieces, direction of the Phaco tip should be away from weak iris
6. Irrigation-aspiration of the epinucleus and cortex which is behind the floppy iris should be removed at last, which avoids catching of the iris during surgery
7. Intraocular lens implantation avoid pressure on the bag which may be weak in these cases.

IMMATURE CATARACT WITH FLOPPY IRIS (FIGS 2A AND B)

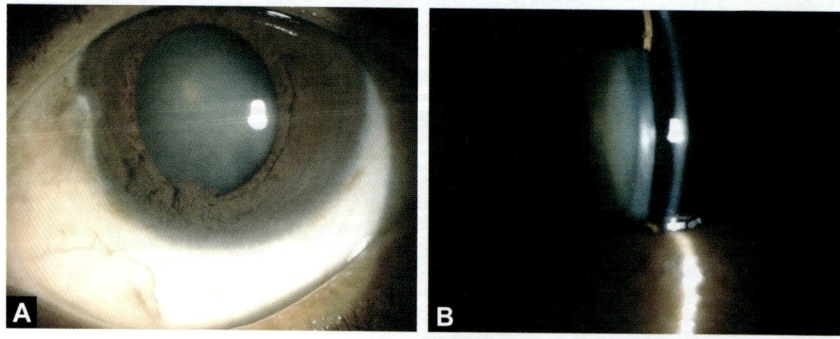

Figs 2A and B (A) Gross view, (B) Slit view

Slit Lamp Examination

Gross View

1. Immature cataract
2. Floppy iris at 6 to 7 o'clock position.

Slit View

1. All layers of the lens are seen
2. Grade 2 dense nucleus
3. Adequate size nucleus means both edges of the nucleus are seen within pupillary area.

Advice

One can go ahead with Phaco surgery easily taking all the precautions mentioned above.

MATURE CATARACT WITH FLOPPY IRIS (FIGS 3A AND B)

Slit Lamp Examination

Gross View

1. Mature cataract
2. Floppy iris at 5 to 6 o'clock.

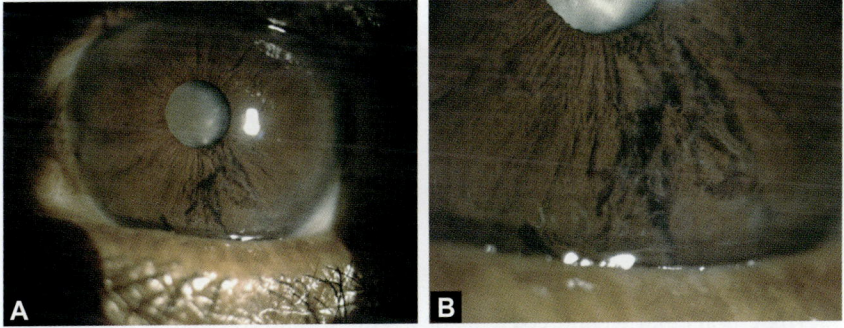

Figs 3A and B (A) Gross view, (B) Magnified view

Advice

1. Phaco surgery can be possible after well dilatation of pupil
2. Sometimes Phaco surgery is unpredictable and conversion to SICS/ECCE is a wise decision.

CATARACT AND FLOPPY IRIS WITH HAZY CORNEA (FIGS 4A TO C)

Slit Lamp Examination

Gross View

1. Hard cataract
2. Hazy cornea
3. Floppy iris from 5 to 7 o'clock, strands of iris directing towards center indicating iris is more fragile.

Slit View

1. All layers of the lens are seen
2. Grade 3 dense nucleus
3. Strands of iris seen inferiorly over the nucleus, 4 PSC element is also seen.

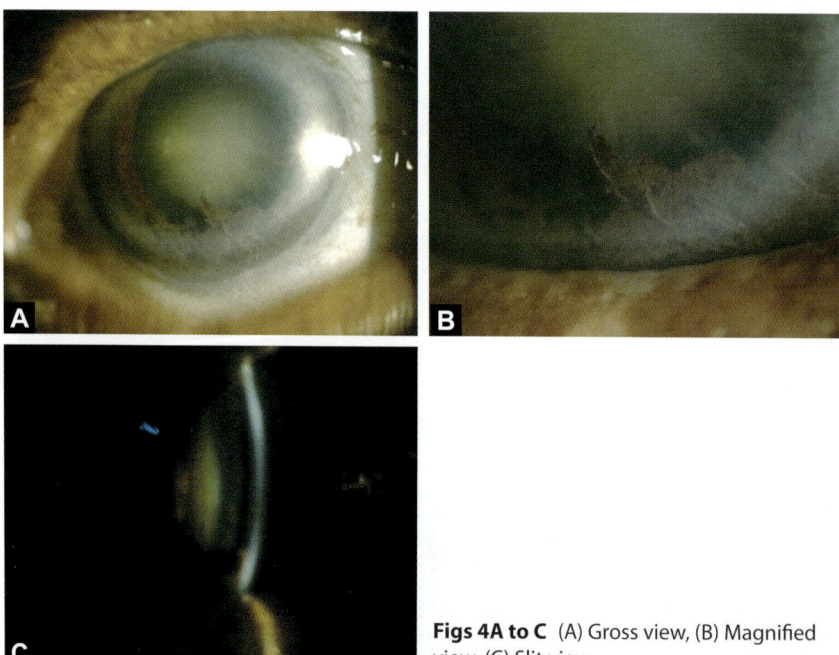

Figs 4A to C (A) Gross view, (B) Magnified view, (C) Slit view

Advice

1. Phaco surgery is advisable
2. High molecular weight viscoelastic agents should be used to keep the iris away
3. Capsulorhexis should be small
4. Trench should be small and should be done cautiously as strands of iris can be caught and causing more damage to the tissue.

NEARLY MATURE CATARACT WITH UNDILATED PUPIL (FIG. 5)

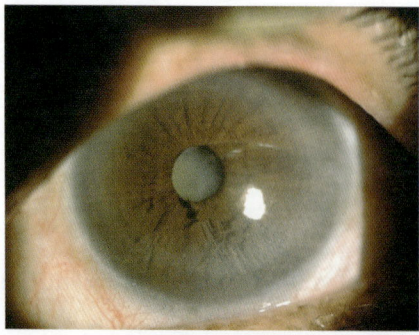

Fig. 5 Gross view

Slit Lamp Examination

Gross View

1. Nearly mature cataract with undilated pupil
2. Floppy iris at 5 to 6 o'clock position.
   - *Significance—after dilatation of pupil, one can miss the size and the location of floppy iris or even presence of floppy iris also.*
   - *It is very important practice to see the cataract cases in undilated position also.*

KEY NOTE
In floppy iris syndrome, avoiding further injury to the iris is the most important factor to be considered during surgery.

Chapter 30

Cataract with Glaucoma

INTRODUCTION

1. This is a very common association noticed in cataract practice.
2. Many times combined surgery (Cataract extraction and glaucoma filtration surgery), cataract extraction or filtering surgery is needed. All these varies from case-to-case and type of cataract and glaucoma.
3. Other anatomical structures like cornea, anterior chamber depth, iris structure, pupil size variation and then finally type of cataract and its detail anatomy will assist to take decision for better visual outcome.

IMMATURE CATARACT WITH GLAUCOMA (FIGS 1A AND B)

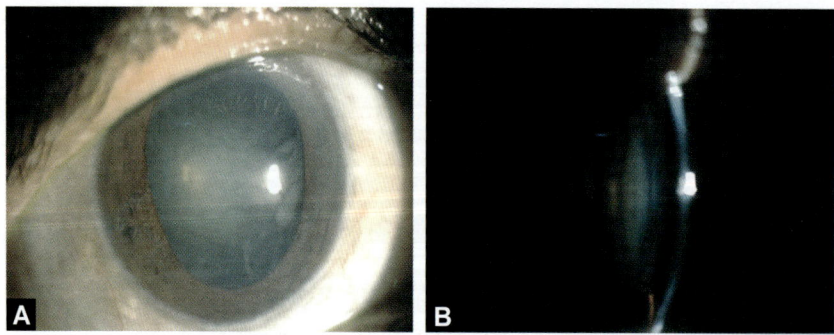

Figs 1A and B (A) Gross view, (B) Slit view

Slit Lamp Examination

Gross View

1. Immature cataract
2. Iris is friable at 8 o'clock position which is sign of previous attacks of glaucoma.

Chapter 30: Cataract with Glaucoma

Slit View

1. All layers of the lens are seen
2. Grade 2 dense nucleus
3. Adequate size of the nucleus
4. Anterior chamber depth is normal (not very shallow).

Advice

Cataract can be easily managed by Phaco surgery along with glaucoma management.

IMMATURE CATARACT AND PERIPHERAL IRIDOTOMY WITH GLAUCOMA (FIGS 2A AND B)

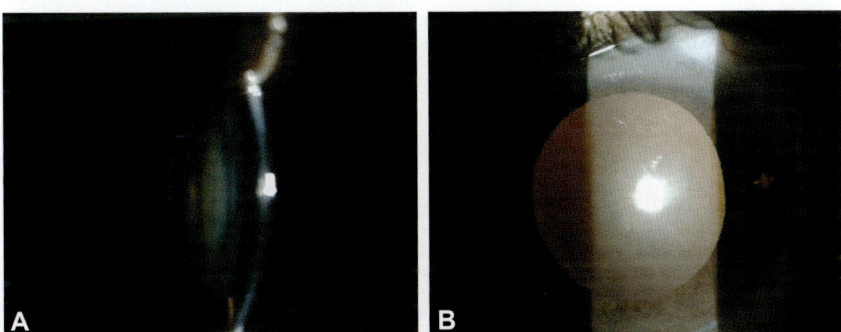

Figs 2A and B (A) Gross view, (B) Retroillumination

Slit Lamp Examination

Gross View

1. Immature cataract.
2. Peripheral iridotomy seen at 3'o clock position.
3. In retroillumination—peripheral iridotomy is clearly visible as a red glow which means it is patent.

Slit View

1. All layers of the lens are seen
2. Grade 2 dense nucleus
3. Adequate size of the nucleus.

Advice

Phaco surgery is easy.

CENTRAL DENSE CATARACT WITH GLAUCOMA (FIG. 3)

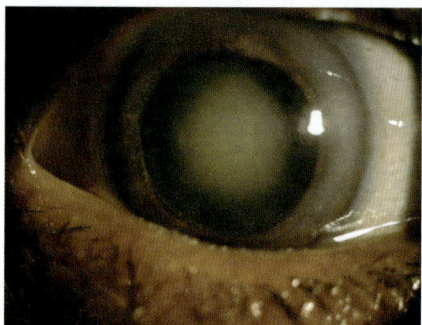

Fig. 3 Gross view

Slit Lamp Examination

Gross View

1. Dense cataract
2. Pupil is adequately dialated
3. Sphincter of iris is damaged due to previous attacks of glaucoma.

Advice

Phaco surgery can be performed.

CATARACT WITH PSEUDOEXFOLIATION AND GLAUCOMA (FIGS 4A AND B)

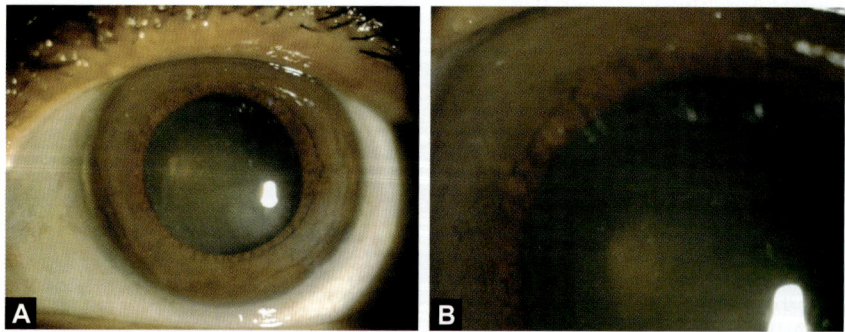

Figs 4A and B (A) Gross view, (B) Slit view

Slit Lamp Examination

Gross View

1. Cataract associated with pseudoexfoliation

2. Mid-dilated pupil
3. Cornea is hazy peripherally.

Advice

Cataract can be managed by Phaco surgery easily with minimum intrabag manipulation.

CATARACT WITH NARROW ANGLE GLAUCOMA (FIG. 5)

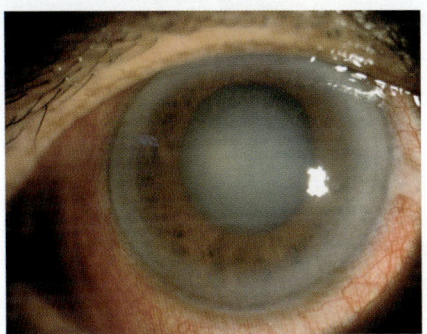

Fig. 5 Gross view

Slit Lamp Examination

Gross View

1. Congested eye
2. Corneal edema
3. Mid-dilated pupil
4. Shallow anterior chamber
5. Immature cataract

Advice

1. Glaucoma management first followed by cataract management
2. Phaco surgery is not very easy due to shallow anterior chamber with cataract.

CATARACT WITH STATUS POST-GLAUCOMA SURGERY (FIGS 6A AND B)

Slit Lamp Examination

Gross View

1. Immature cataract
2. Mid-dilated pupil
3. Filtering bleb is flat.

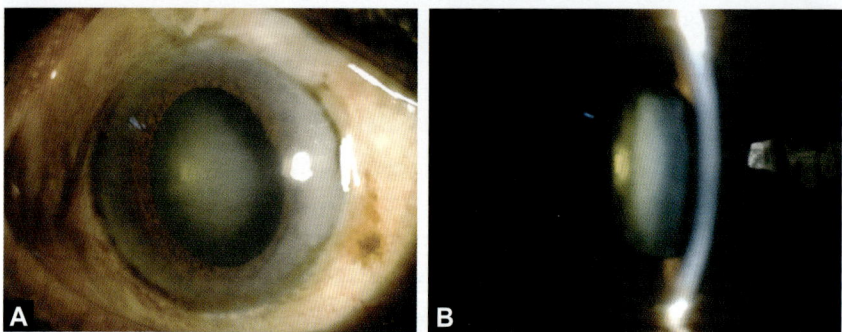

Figs 6A and B (A) Gross view, (B) Slit view

Slit View

1. All layers of the lens are seen
2. Grade 2 to 3 density nucleus
3. Adequate size nucleus
4. Anterior chamber is shallow.

Advice

Repeat filtering surgery with cataract extraction by Phaco surgery or ECCE.

KEY NOTE

Decision of the surgery either cataract extraction, glaucoma surgery, or combined cataract and glaucoma surgery and depends on AC depth, IOP, type of glaucoma and condition of the lens.

Chapter 31

Cataract with Iris Coloboma

INTRODUCTION

1. Defect in the iris is seen inferiorly. It may be partially present or completely absent. It can be associated with zonular weakness, zonular absence and sometimes defect in the lens also.
2. Phaco surgery can be done in these cases with consideration of zonular dehiscence inferiorly.
3. Incision can be taken temporally. In superior incision direction of the trench should be oblique so that it remains away from area of dehiscence.
4. During division equal pressure is mandatory which can be managed by prechopper like instrument.
5. Hold and lift should be very slow and one should avoid pull on dehiscence area.
6. Viscoelastic should be injected from the side port before Phaco probe is taken out to keep the bag inflated after removal of small pieces.
7. Irrigation-aspiration is crucial.
8. Consideration of foldable as well as polymethylmethacrylate (PMMA) intraocular lens should be there.
9. Capsular tension ring may be needed in many situations.

IRIS COLOBOMA WITH IMMATURE CATARACT (FIGS 1A TO C)

Slit Lamp Examination

Gross View

Iris coloboma with immature cataract.

Slit View

1. Iris coloboma confirmed.
2. Defect in the lens was noticed inferiorly (Fig. 1C).
3. Grade 2 dense nucleus.
4. Small size of nucleus.

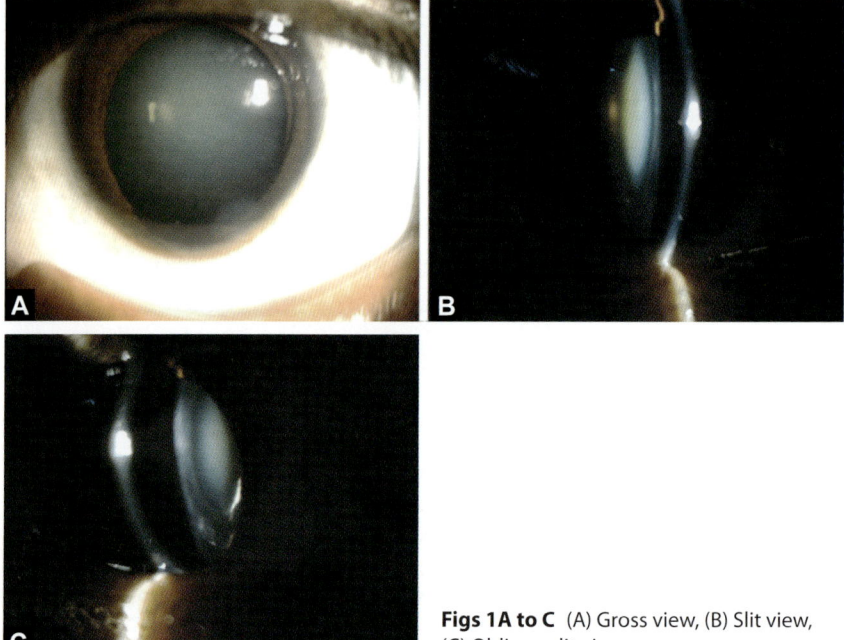

Figs 1A to C (A) Gross view, (B) Slit view, (C) Oblique slit view

Advice

Phaco surgery can be done.

IRIS COLOBOMA WITH DENSE CATARACT (FIGS 2A AND B)

Slit Lamp Examination

Gross View

Iris coloboma with dense cataract.

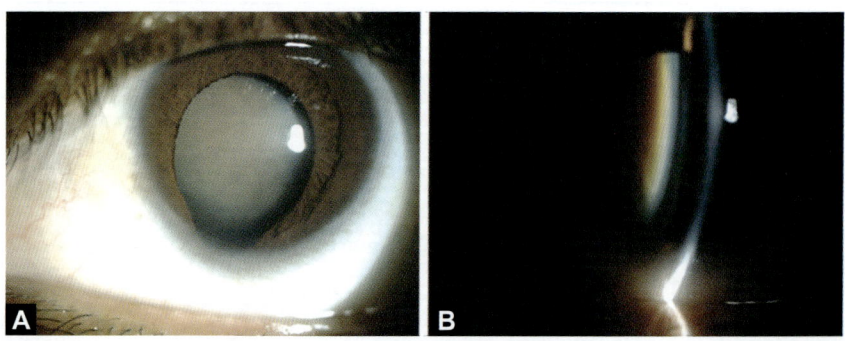

Figs 2A and B (A) Gross view, (B) Slit view

Slit View

1. All layers of the lens are seen.
2. Grade 4 to 5 dense nucleus.
3. Long length of nucleus.

Advice

1. Phaco surgery can be managed with difficulty.
2. Surgeon should be ready for conversion to small incision cataract surgery (SICS)/extracapsular cataract extraction (ECCE).

IRIS COLOBOMA WITH SOFT CATARACT (FIGS 3A AND B)

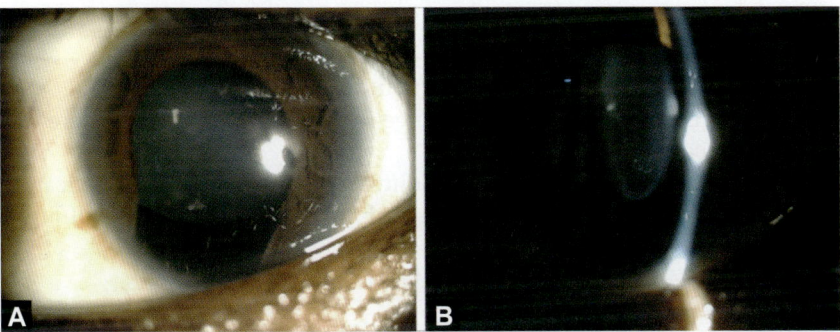

Figs 3A and B (A) Gross view, (B) Slit view

Slit Lamp Examination

Gross View

1. Iris coloboma with soft cataract.
2. Inferior iris defect is very large.
3. Absence of zonules noticed at the same site.

Slit View

1. Very soft cataract.
2. All layers of the lens are seen.
3. *Lens is globular in shape which confirms absence of zonules inferiorly.*

Advice

1. Capsulorhexis is difficult.
2. Capsular tension ring (CTR) is needed.

KEY NOTE
This is one of the difficult situations as the pupil is downdrawn and associated with abnormal zonular condition.

Chapter 32

Cataract with Micro-ophthalmos

INTRODUCTION

1. By definition all the anatomical structures are smaller than normal.
2. Cataract extraction is a real challenge in these cases. Difficulties are due to microcornea, shallow AC, etc.
3. This is noticed in young age. This condition is one of the contraindication to put intraocular lens (IOL) (one can think of special design of IOL).

MATURE CATARACT WITH MICRO-OPHTHALMOS (FIG. 1)

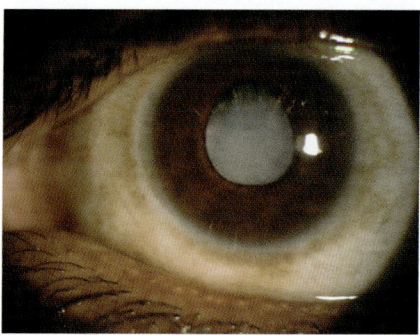

Fig. 1 Gross view

Slit Lamp Examination

Gross View

1. Mature cataract with micro-ophthalmos.
2. Small cornea.
3. Shallow AC.

CENTRAL CATARACT WITH MICRO-OPHTHALMOS (FIG. 2)

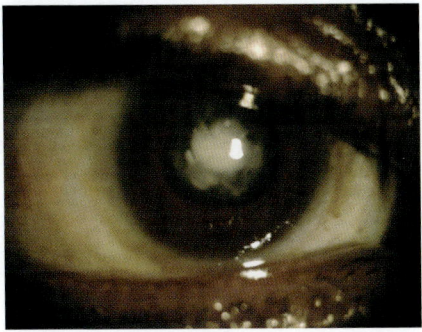

Fig. 2 Gross view

Slit Lamp Examination

Gross View

1. Small cornea.
2. Shallow AC.
3. Central cataract.

Advice

Cataract surgery is difficult.

KEY NOTE
Intraocular lens implantation is contraindicated.

Chapter 33

Cataract with Vitreous Opacities

INTRODUCTION

1. Association of cataract with vitreous opacities is not uncommon as both conditions are present in old age.
2. Surgeons should not take decision in hurry in such cases.
3. Good counseling is important.
4. In management, red glow is impaired so there is difficulty during capsulorhexis, trench, removal of small pieces, irrigation-aspiration and foldable intraocular lens (IOL) implantation.
5. Due to visualization problem, chances of posterior capsule rupture (PCR) are quiet common during surgery.

DIFFUSE CAT WITH VITREOUS OPACITIES (FIGS 1A AND B)

Slit Lamp Examination

Gross View

Diffuse cataract with vitreous opacities.

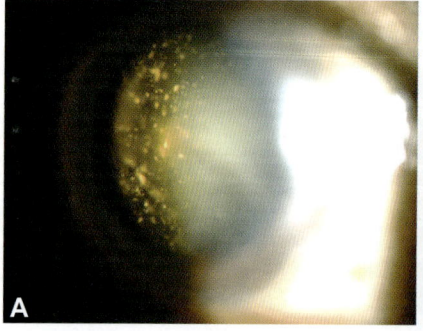
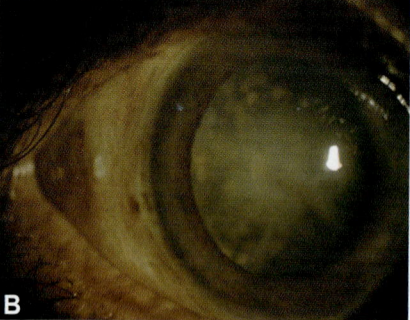

Figs 1A and B Gross view: (A) Light focused posteriorly at vitreous plane, (B) Light focused at lens plane

VITREOUS OPACITIES WITH SOFT CATARACT (FIGS 2A AND B)

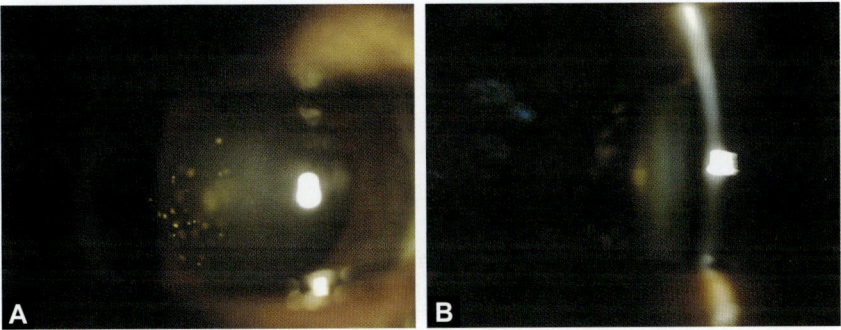

Figs 2A and B (A) Gross view, (B) Slit view

Slit Lamp Examination

Gross View

1. Very soft cataract.
2. Vitreous opacities seen.

Slit View

1. All layers of the lens are seen.
2. Soft cataract.
3. Adequate size and thin nucleus, with PSC element is also seen.

Advice

1. Phaco surgery is easy.
2. Precaution during trench as it is thin nucleus.
3. One should take all precautions which mentioned before.

CATARACT WITH VITREOUS OPACITIES (FIG. 3)

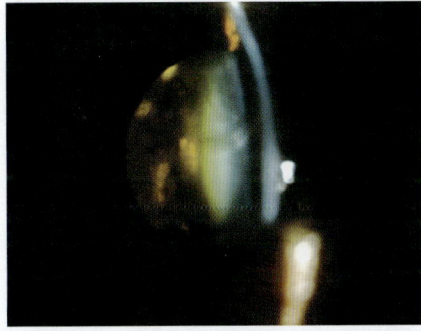

Fig. 3 Slit view

Slit Lamp Examination

Slit View

1. All layers of the lens are seen
2. Grade 3 nucleus
3. Adequate size of nucleus
4. Vitreous opacities are seen distinctly.

Advice

Phaco surgery is more easy with all precautions mentioned earlier than previous case due to adequate density and size of nucleus.

KEY NOTE

Most important fact in cataract with vitreous opacity is that, nucleus management steps like trench, division, hold and lift, are easy but are the main difficulty in removal of small pieces, (especially last pieces), irrigation-aspiration and foldable IOL implantation is due to empty bag and then these vitreous opacities will seen prominently which make visualization difficult.

Chapter 34

Cataract with Pterygium

INTRODUCTION

1. This is a very common condition seen in daily practice.
2. Another considerable factor is size of pterygium, whether it is from one side or both sides and area of pupil covered by pterygium which is important to modify the steps of surgery.
3. Visualization is hampered in such cases.
4. Space for surgical steps is restricted as cornea is covered by pterygium.
5. *Issue of astigmatism is unanswered in such cases.*
6. Ideal way is to remove the pterygium first followed by cataract extraction after few weeks. But there are some situations where one should consider removing the cataract first. Following discussion is related to that.

CATARACT WITH PTERYGIUM (FIGS 1A AND B)

Slit Lamp Examination

Gross View

Central dense cataract with pterygium covering up to the center of pupil from one side.

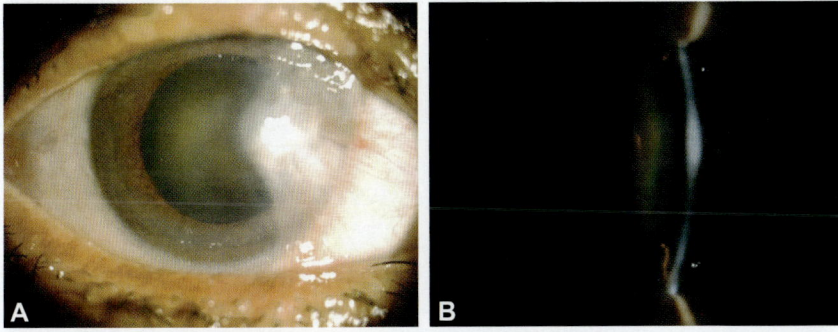

Figs 1A and B (A) Gross view, (B) Slit view

Slit View

1. Grade 3 dense nucleus.
2. Adequate size nucleus.

IMMATURE CATARACT WITH PTERYGIUM (FIGS 2A AND B)

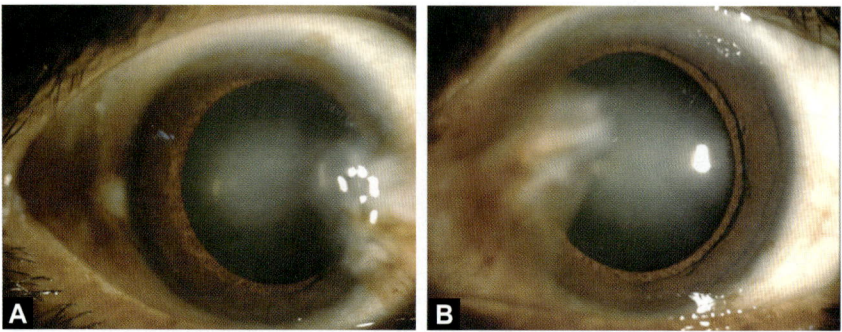

Figs 2A and B Gross view

Slit Lamp Examination

Gross View

1. Immature cataract.
2. Pterygium from one side.

HARD CATARACT WITH EARLY PTERYGIUM (FIGS 3A AND B)

Slit Lamp Examination

Gross View

1. Hard cataract.
2. Mid-dilated pupil.
3. Early pterygium.

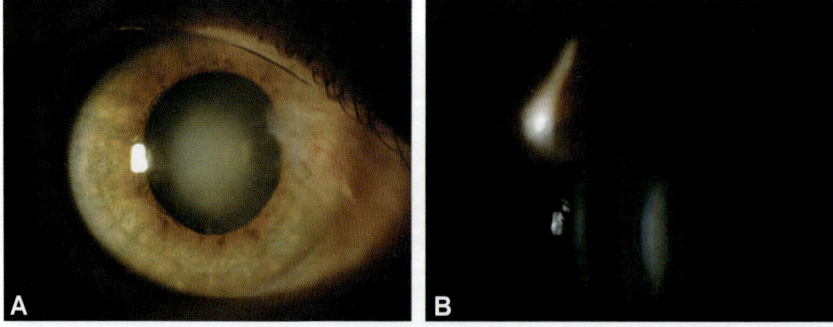

Figs 3A and B (A) Gross view, (B) Slit view

Slit View

1. Grade 3 dense nucleus.
2. Small size of nucleus.

Advice (Figs 1 to 3)

Phaco surgery is easy in all these situations with some modifications.
1. Side port incision can be avoided on pterygium or should be done away from pterygium.
2. One can do side port through pterygium followed by cauterization of bleeders.
3. Capsulorhexis should be done in the visible part of pupillary area that means it should not be done blindly behind the pterygium or it can be done behind the pterygium area by tilting the eyeball.
4. In trench, many times one has to do paracentral trench.
5. Hold and lift should be done in half part of nucleus which is visible.
6. Removal of small pieces should be done under visualization.
7. Irrigation-aspiration is difficult behind the pterygium area and should be done cautiously.

HARD NUCLEUS WITH ADVANCED PTERYGIUM (FIGS 4A AND B)

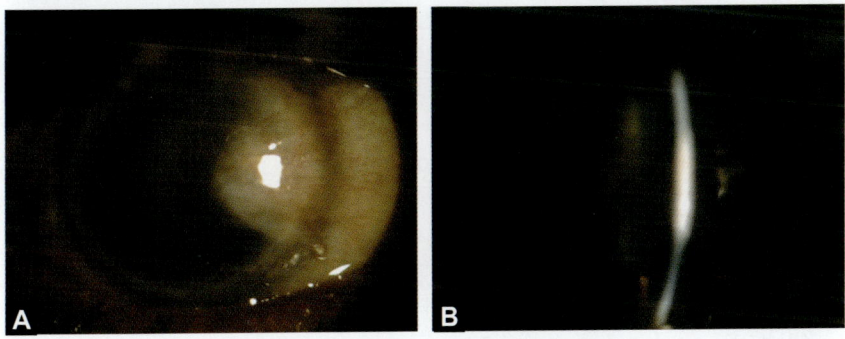

Figs 4A and B (A) Gross view, (B) Slit view

Slit Lamp Examination

Gross View

1. Hard nucleus with advanced pterygium.
2. Hazy cornea.

Slit View

1. Grade 4 dense nucleus.
2. Central shadow of pterygium on nucleus noticed.

Advice

1. Difficult to do phaco surgery.
2. Difficulty is due to advanced pterygium, hazy cornea with big size dense nucleus.
3. Sometimes conversion to small incision cataract surgery (SICS) or extracapsular cataract extraction (ECCE) can be considered.

HARD CATARACT WITH PTERYGIUM ON BOTH SIDES (FIGS 5A AND B)

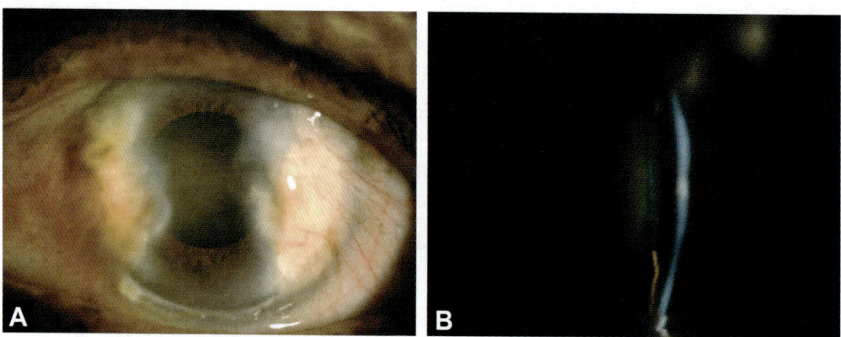

Figs 5A and B (A) Gross view, (B) Slit view

Slit Lamp Examination

Gross View

1. Hard cataract with pterygium on both sides.
2. Cornea is hazy.

Slit View

1. Irregularity of cornea is confirmed by irregular corneal slit with shadow on lens.
2. Hazy cornea.
3. Grade 4 dense nucleus.
4. Big size nucleus.

Advice

1. Phaco surgery as that of hard cataract management with some modifications.
2. Capsulorhexis should be vertically oval.
3. Trech and division can be done easily under visualization.
4. Hold and lift of each half of nucleus can be done by rotating the nucleus at 6 o'clock position.

5. Difficulty of irrigation-aspiration of epinucleus and cortex has been increased due to pterygium on both sides.

Advice

One should think any time to convert to SICS or ECCE as this not very simple case.

CATARACT WITH PTERYGIUM ON BOTH SIDES (FIGS 6A AND B)

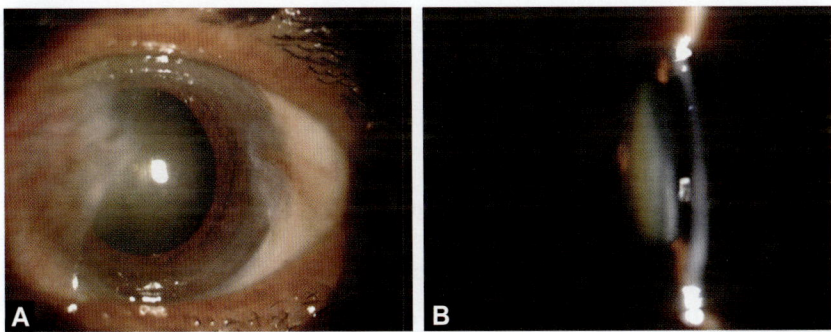

Figs 6A and B (A) Gross view, (B) Slit view

Slit Lamp Examination

Gross View

1. Cataract with pterygium on both sides.
2. One advanced and one small.
3. Cornea is relatively clear.

Slit View

1. Grade 3 dense nucleus.
2. Adequate size of nucleus.

Advice

Steps of the Phaco surgery are relatively simple than previous case.

KEY NOTE
In these cases, area of Phaco surgery is restricted than normal due to hampered visualization by pterygium.

Chapter 35

Cataract with Mooren's Ulcer

INTRODUCTION

1. Mooren's ulcer is peripheral degeneration of cornea.
2. This condition is commonly found in old age, so association of this condition with cataract is quiet common.

Difficulty in the management in these cases are as follows:
1. Hazy cornea.
2. Peripheral thinning of the cornea particularly inferiorly.
3. Inflamed eye which may be painful.
4. Conjunctiva, sclera and cornea may be fragile and thin.

IMMATURE CATARACT WITH MOOREN'S ULCER (FIG. 1)

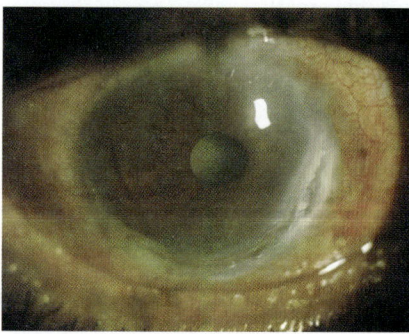

Fig. 1 Gross view

Slit Lamp Examination

Gross View

1. Mooren's ulcer with inflamed eye.
2. Immature cataract.
3. Cornea is hazy.

Advice

1. Phaco surgery can be done.
2. Many times conversion to small incision cataract surgery (SICS) or extracapsular cataract extraction (ECCE) is a wise decision.

KEY NOTE
Difficulty for surgical management in these cases is due to hazy cornea and inflamed eye.

Chapter 36

Cataract in Post-radial Keratotomy Case

INTRODUCTION

1. These are usually young patients.
2. Cataract is soft.
3. Cataract management is not difficult in these cases.
4. *Most crucial factor is IOL power calculation.*
5. Some modification in cataract procedure is also needed.

CATARACT IN POST-RADIAL KERATOTOMY (FIGS 1A TO D)

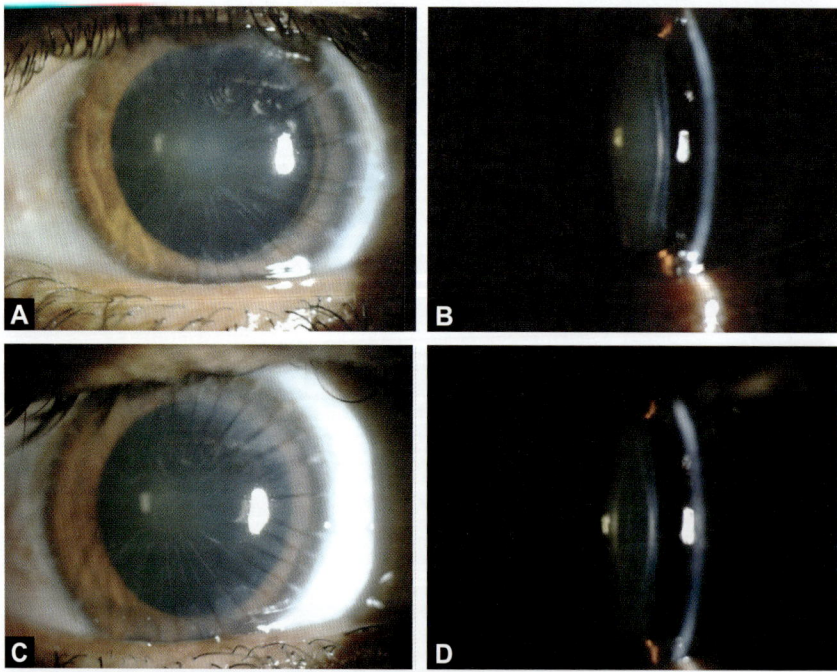

Figs 1A to D (A, C) Gross view, (B, D) Slit view

Slit Lamp Examination

Gross View

1. Dilated pupil.
2. Soft cataract.
3. Marks of radial keratotomy clearly seen on cornea.

Slit View

1. Layers of the lens are well-defined.
2. Anterior chamber is deep.
3. Grade 1 soft nuclear cataract (Fig. 1B).
4. In other eye, there is no nucleus (Fig. 1D).

Advice

1. One can do Phaco surgery easily with some modifications.
2. Limbal incision is the choice which can be performed between the two markings of radial keratotomy.
3. In capsulorhexis, one can avoid trypan blue like solution in such cases as it may stain the cornea which can hamper the view. High molecular weight viscoelastics are helpful for capsulorhexis as well as protection to corneal endothelium.
4. Further management is as that of soft cataract.
5. Most important point of consideration is when Phaco probe or irrigation-aspiration cannula is in the eye, with the force of irrigating fluid there may be chances of gaping at the site of radial keratotomy incision.

KEY NOTE
Most important difficulty in such cases is visualization and hypotony.

Chapter 37

Cataract in Post-penetrating Keratoplasty Case

INTRODUCTION

1. This is one of the challenging situation to do cataract surgery.
2. Disturbing points may be hazy cornea, scaring of keratoplasty surgery.

IMMATURE CATARACT IN POST-PENETRATING KERATOPLASTY CASE (FIGS 1A AND B)

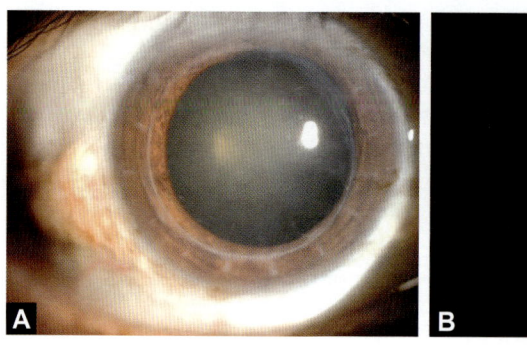
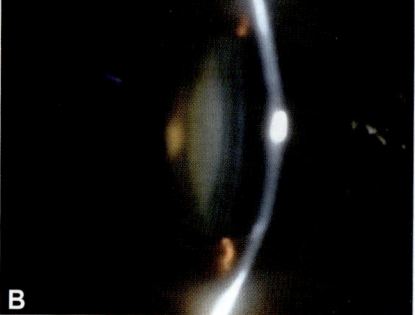

Figs 1A and B (A) Gross view, (B) Slit view

Slit Lamp Examination

Gross View

1. Immature cataract in post-penetrating keratoplasty case.
2. Donor cornea is clear.
3. Pupil is adequately dilated.

Slit View

1. All layers of the lens are seen.
2. Grade 2 nucleus density.

3. Adequate size of nucleus.
4. Posterior subcapsular cataract (PSC) is seen.

Advice

Phaco surgery can be performed easily.

KEY NOTE
Difficulty in such condition is due to visualization and astigmatic consideration is unanswered.

Chapter 38

Cataract in Post-trabeculectomy Cases

INTRODUCTION

1. This is one of the challenging situations for cataract surgeon.
2. Following are the difficulties in these situations:
   - Hazy cornea
   - Location and size of bleb
   - AC depth which may be shallow or uneven
   - Pupil is not fully dilated
   - Suspicious zonular weakness
   - Only important criteria is to treat these cases is size and hardness of nucleus and accordingly surgeon can take decision of doing Phaco surgery or not.

DENSE CATARACT WITH FILTERING BLEB (FIGS 1A AND B)

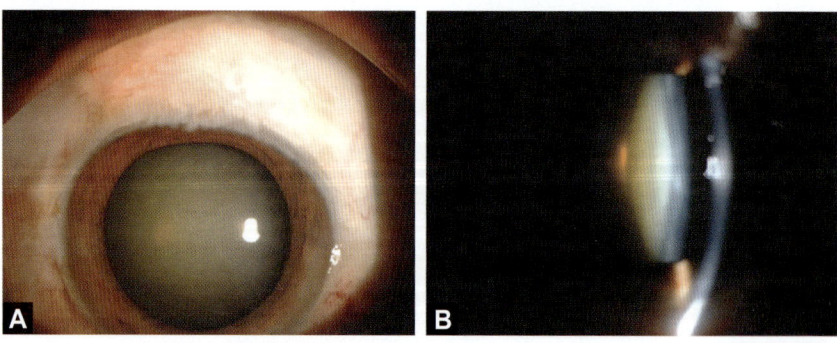

Figs 1A and B (A) Gross view, (B) Slit view

Slit Lamp Examination

Gross View

1. Bleb seen at 12 o'clock.
2. Dense cataract.
3. Well dilated pupil.

Slit View

1. All layers of the lens are seen.
2. Grade 3 dense nucleus.
3. Adequate size of nucleus.

Advice

1. Phaco surgery can be done easily.
2. Incision should be clear corneal or temporal approach can be considered.
3. Intrabag manipulations should be minimum as zonules may be compromised.

DENSE CATARACT WITH ENCROACHMENT OF FILTERING BLEB ON CORNEA (FIGS 2A AND B)

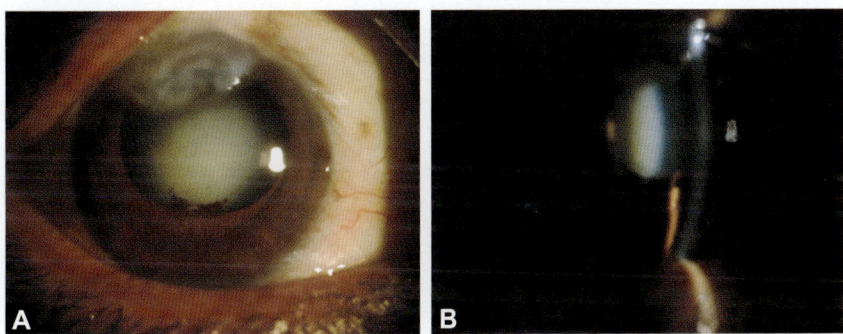

Figs 2A and B (A) Gross view, (B) Slit view

Slit Lamp Examination

Gross View

1. Anterior encroachment of bleb is seen with dense cataract.
2. Semidilated pupil with posterior synechiae.

Slit View

Dense nucleus is confirmed.

Advice

1. Temporal approach for Phaco surgery.
2. Management of small pupil is needed.
3. Capsulorhexis should be of adequate size.
4. In trench, energy used more than needed to avoid pressure on zonules.

5. In division, avoid uneven pressure for division of nucleus. Division with the prechopper will be preferable.
6. Hold and lift on half part of the nucleus should be slow to avoid pull on zonules.
7. Rest of the steps of Phaco surgery are as routine.

KEY NOTE

Consideration of the zonular weakness and anterior chamber depth is important.

Chapter 39

Cataract in Young Age

INTRODUCTION

1. This is unusual cataract but now a days this is quite common condition seen in day to day practice.
2. Cataract in young patients may be secondary to diabetes, steroid induced, developmental, trauma or sometimes occupational hazards.
3. Management of these cases is not easy as young patients are always anxious. Positive pressure will be there in many cases.
4. *Capsulorhexis is challenging due to elasticity of capsule.*
5. Soft cataract management is another challenging factor related to nuclear management and irrigation-aspiration.
6. *Sometimes challenges in young patients are due to discrimination between age criteria and nuclear density and size. In other words cataract in young patients may be associated with big size or hard nucleus.*

IMMATURE CATARACT (FIGS 1A AND B)

Slit Lamp Examination

Gross View

Immature cataract with central dense nucleus.

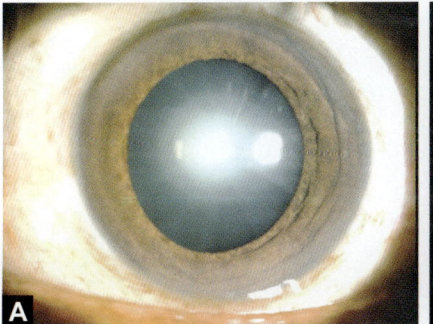 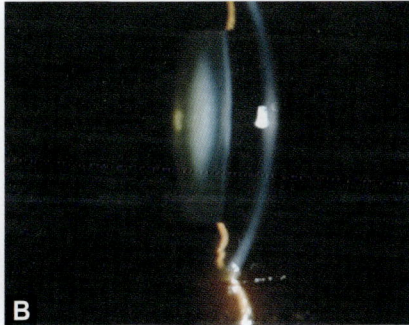

Figs 1A and B (A) Gross view, (B) Slit view

Slit View

1. All layers of the lens are seen.
2. Small size nucleus.
3. Grade 2 dense nucleus.

Advice

Phaco surgery is easy.

VERY SOFT CATARACT (FIG. 2)

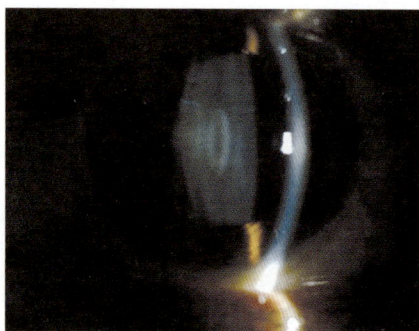

Fig. 2 Slit view

Slit Lamp Examination

Slit View

Central ring like appearance of cataract, surrounded by cortical cataract.

Advice

1. Viscoexpression of nucleus is method of choice.
2. Irrigation-aspiration is always crucial in such cases.

DIFFUSE CATARACT (FIGS 3A AND B)

Slit Lamp Examination

Gross View

1. Diffuse cataract.
2. Mid-dilated pupil.

Slit View

1. All layers of the lens are seen.
2. Cortical cataract with PSC is seen.

Chapter 39: Cataract in Young Age

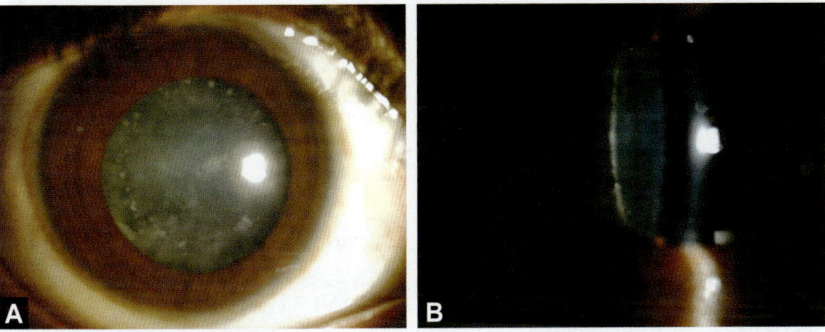

Figs 3A and B (A) Gross view, (B) Slit view

Advice

Viscoexpression of soft tissue and irrigation-aspiration, will complete the procedure.

CENTRAL CATARACT (FIGS 4A AND B)

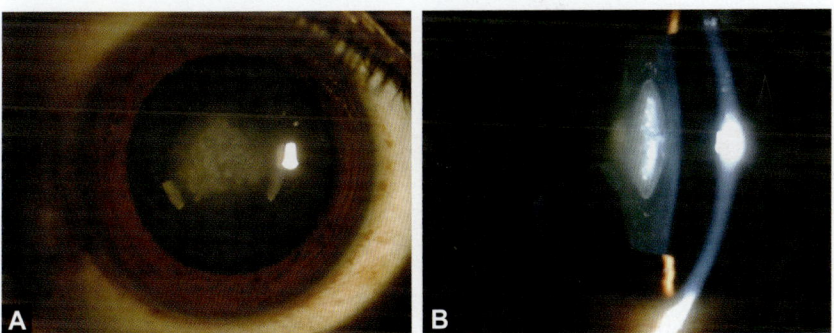

Figs 4A and B (A) Gross view, (B) Slit view

Slit Lamp Examination

Gross View

1. Central dense cataract is surrounded by diffuse opacity of lens.
2. Soft cataract.

Slit View

1. All layers of the lens are seen.
2. Central dense nucleus confirmed.
3. Diffuse lens haze is also noticed.

Advice

1. Viscoexpression of nucleus and epinucleus is the choice.
2. Irrigation-aspiration should be done cautiously.

CORTICAL CATARACT (FIGS 5A AND B)

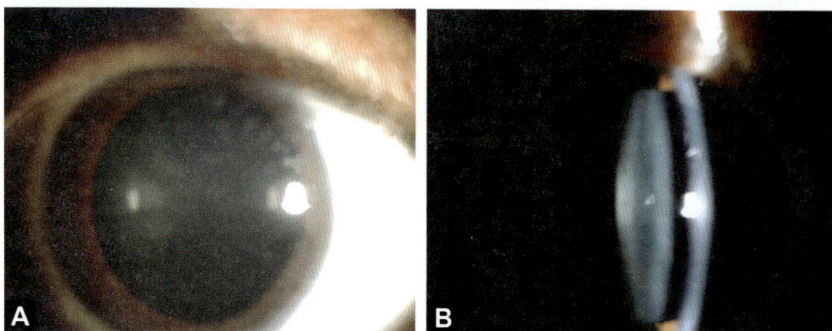

Figs 5A and B (A) Gross view, (B) Slit view

Slit Lamp Examination

Gross View

1. Cortical cataract.
2. *One can label this case as a normal lens haze also.*

Slit View

Confirms cortical cataract with no nucleus.

Advice

Viscoexpression of soft tissue and irrigation-aspiration is helpful in this case.

IMMATURE CATARACT (FIGS 6A AND B)

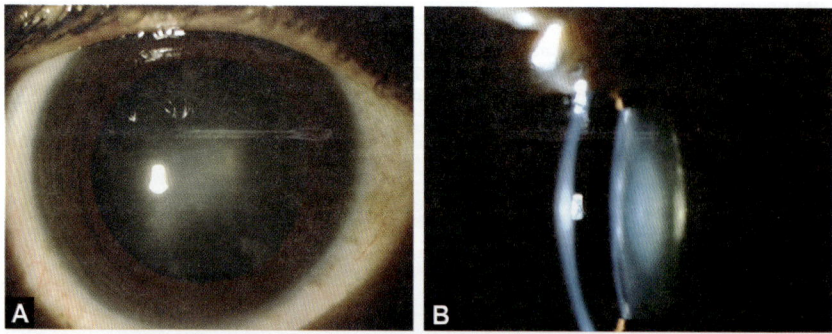

Figs 6A and B (A) Gross view, (B) Slit view

Slit Lamp Examination

Gross View

1. Central nuclear cataract.
2. Cortical cataract.

Slit View

1. All the layers of lens are cataractous, i.e. ASC, cortical, central nuclear and PSC.
2. *This is unusual variety of cataract in young patients where all the layers are involved.*

Advice

1. Visco expression of nucleus management is unique technique in such cases.
2. Irrigation-aspiration should be done with patience.

CENTRAL DENSE CATARACT (FIGS 7A AND B)

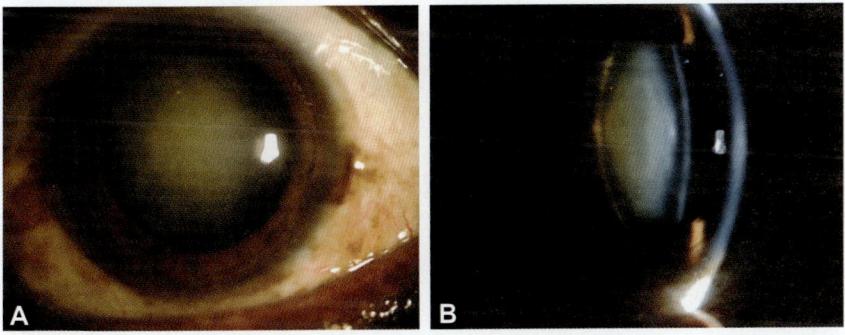

Figs 7A and B (A) Gross view, (B) Slit view

Slit Lamp Examination

Gross View

1. Central dense cataract.
2. Semidilated pupil.

Slit View

1. All layers of the lens are seen clearly.
2. *Grade 2 to 3 density of endonucleus which is well demarcated and outlined by soft part of nucleus which is grade 2 dense. PSC is also seen.*

Advice

Stop and chop technique of Phaco surgery is preferred.

VARIETIES OF CATARACT IN YOUNG PATIENT (FIGS 8A AND B)

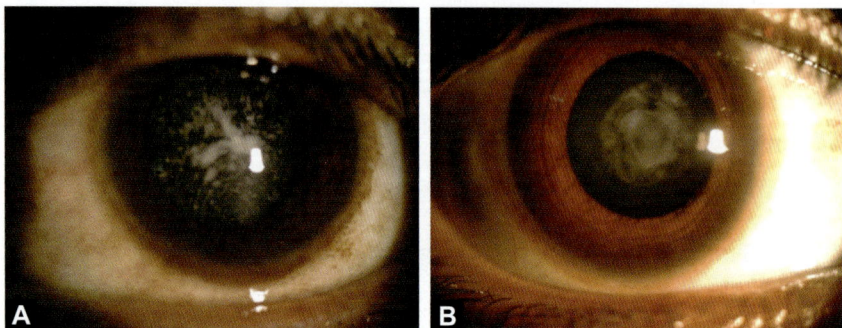

Figs 8A and B Gross view

Slit Lamp Examination

Gross View

Central cataract seen in both cases.

Advice

Management in such cases as if in soft variety of cataract.

Key Note
1. *Capsulorhexis is one of the most challenging steps in these cases.*
2. *General anesthesia is needed in many cases.*

Chapter 40

Cataract in Old Age

INTRODUCTION

1. Cataract is usually seen in old age patients.
2. Point of consideration is that hard cataract, soft cataract, mature cataract, pseudoexfoliation cataract associated with very old age, need management accordingly.
3. *One has to remember that we are performing surgery on a weak or unhealthy bag.*

HARD CATARACT (FIGS 1A AND B)

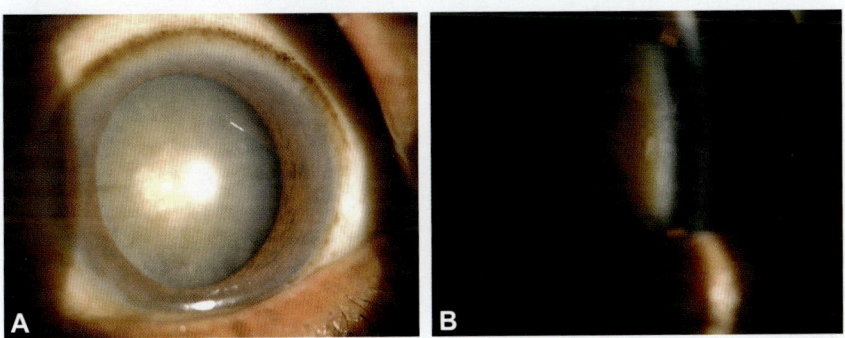

Figs 1A and B (A) Gross view, (B) Slit view

Slit Lamp Examination

Gross view

1. Very hard cataract.
2. Dilated pupil.

Slit View

1. All layers of the lens are seen.
2. Grade 5 to 6 dense nucleus.
3. Big size nucleus.

Advice

1. In old age zonules may be weak, endothelial cell count is less, density of nucleus is more than assumed, overall anatomy is more degenerated.
2. Considering all these factors, one can avoid Phaco and do small incision cataract surgery (SICS)/extracapsular cataract extraction (ECCE).

SOFT CATARACT (FIGS 2A AND B)

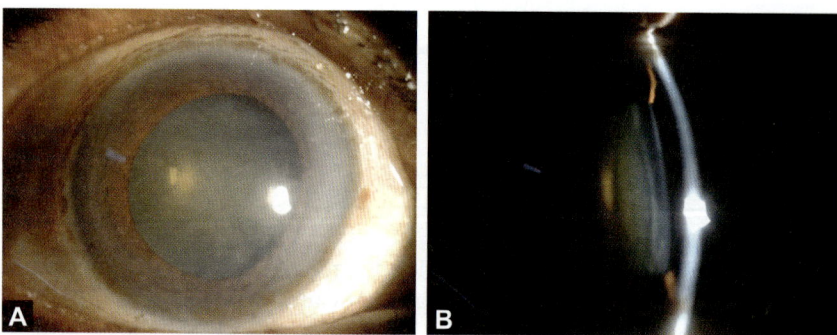

Figs 2A and B (A) Gross view, (B) Slit view

Slit Lamp Examination

Gross View

1. Immature cataract.
2. Pupil is not fully dilated.
3. Cornea is hazy.

Slit View

1. All layers of the lens are seen.
2. Soft cataract.
3. Big size nucleus.

Advice

Soft cataract in old age is always difficult as these are the sticky cataract. But one can perform phaco easily in these cases.

KEY NOTE
Very hard cataract and soft cataract in old age is difficult to manage.

Chapter 41

Cataract with Uneven Anterior Chamber

INTRODUCTION

1. Adherent leukoma is very common condition where iris is adherent to the cornea which is already opacified (leukoma grade).
2. This condition is associated with different shape and size of pupil and most important considerable factor is *uneven anterior chamber*.

Phaco surgery may be difficult in these situations due to following reasons:
- Hazy view.
- Pupil is not adequately dilated.
- *Phaco fluidics is not usual due to uneven anterior chamber.*
- Chances of iris prolapse is common due to misdirection of current of irrigating fluid.
- Anterior chamber volume is less than normal and is more common in corneal incision.
- *All the steps of nucleus management is different and difficult due to uneven Phaco fluidics.*

BOTH EYES ADHERENT LEUKOMA (FIGS 1A AND B)

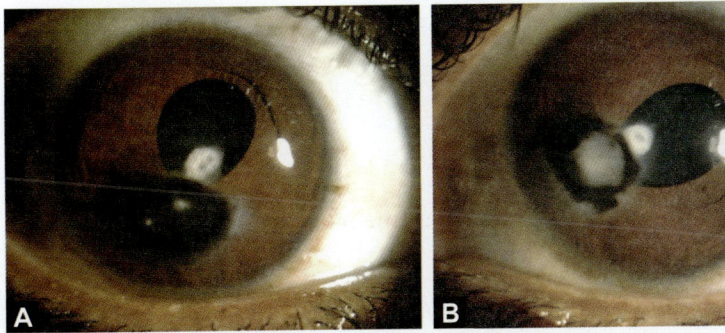

Figs 1A and B Gross view—both eyes

Slit Lamp Examination

Gross View

1. Adherent leukoma with central cataract in both eyes.
2. Tattooing of corneal opacity is noticed.

Advice

1. Phaco surgery can be done with all modification.
2. Pupil needs special management.

ADHERENT LEUKOMA WITH CATARACT (FIGS 2A AND B)

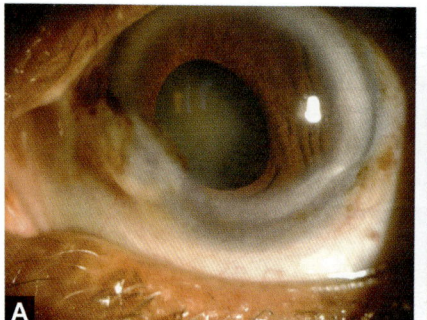 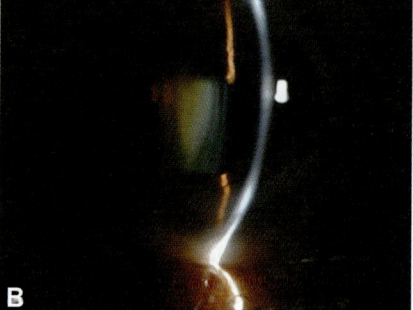

Figs 2A and B (A) Gross view, (B) Slit view

Slit Lamp Examination

Gross View

1. Adherent leukoma with cataract.
2. Dense arcus senilis.

Slit View

1. All layers of the lens are seen.
2. Grade 3 dense cataract.
3. Adequate size of nucleus.

Advice

Phaco surgery can be done after management of pupil.

KEY NOTE
Phaco fluidics is unusual due to uneven anterior chamber.

Chapter 42

Cataract with Wrinkling of Face

INTRODUCTION

1. As patient enters in the outpatient department (OPD), overall examination of the patient as a whole is important. During torch light examination, it is important to examine the skin of the face specifically periocular area is important. *Wrinkling of the face gives an idea about degeneration of the skin. Author has very strong suggestion to correlate this finding with zonular strength of the bag.*
2. Management part depends on this finding. One should avoid excessive intrabag manipulation during Phaco surgery to avoid stress on zonules.

CATARACT WITH WRINKLING OF FACE (FIGS 1A TO D)

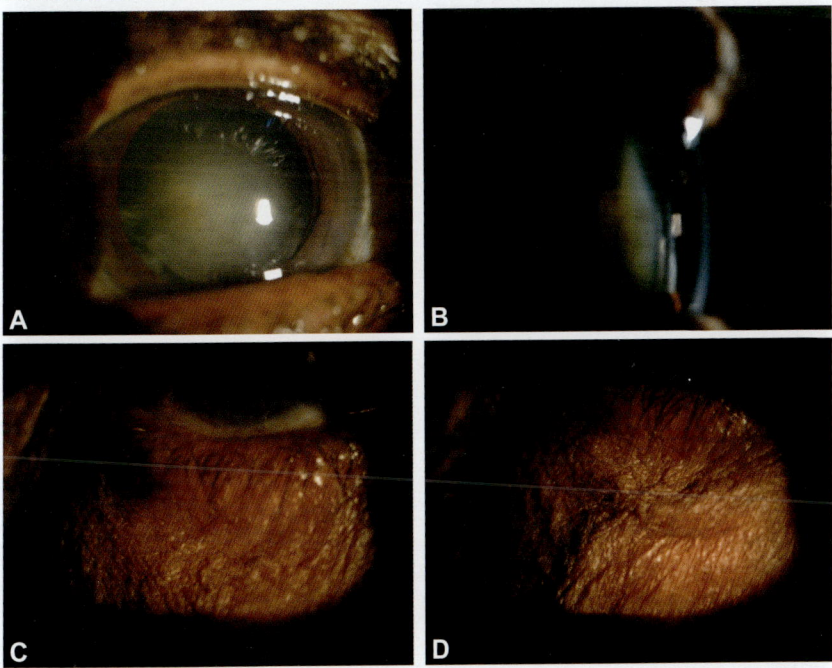

Figs 1A to D (A) Gross view, (B) Slit view, (C and D) Wrinkling of skin in periocular area

Slit Lamp Examination

Gross View

Dense cataract.

Slit View

1. All layers of the lens are seen.
2. Grade 3 dense nucleus.
3. Adequate size nucleus.

Gross View of Periocular Area

Wrinkling of skin seen.

Advice

Phaco surgery is easy with all precautions of not giving pressure on zonules during intrabag manipulation.

KEY NOTE
Consideration of zonular weakness related to wrinkling of the periocular skin is a different way to assess the condition of the lens.

Index

Page numbers followed by f refer to figure

A

Anterior capsule rupture 91
Anterior subcapsular cataract 3, 6, 59, 68, 80

B

Bread crumb appearance 14
Bulky nucleus 48

C

Calcified capsular bag 104
Capsulorhexis 10, 53
Cataract 109
   central 28, 165, 185
      anterior subcapsular 6, 83
      dense 4, 5, 137, 158, 187
      hard 43
      nuclear 28, 187
   cortical 19, 34, 59, 60, 62, 63, 84, 186, 187
      and central posterior subcapsular 87
      and nuclear 28
   dense 57, 81, 139, 140, 158, 180, 194
   diabetic 80
   extraction 156
      extracapsular 103, 137, 172, 175, 190
      intracapsular 106
   in old age 189
   in post-radial keratotomy 176
   in post-trabeculectomized eye 133
   in young age 183
   mature 30, 81, 120, 153
   soft 23, 54, 58, 81, 84, 117, 177, 190
   sticky 152
   subluxated 103
   traumatic 88
   typical diabetic 80
Cataract with
   big size nucleus 55
   central posterior synechiae 89
   corneal opacity and hazy cornea 137
   different shapes of pupil 143
   embedded foreign body in lens 149
   floppy iris syndrome 151
   glaucoma 156, 158
   hyperopia 145
   iris coloboma 161
   micro-ophthalmos 164, 165
   Mooren's ulcer 174
   multiple weak zones 73
   myopia 147
   narrow angle glaucoma 159
   neovascular glaucoma 85, 85f
   pseudoexfoliation 113, 135, 158
   pterygium 169, 173
   shallow anterior chamber 123
   small pupil 129
   small size nucleus 51
   status post-glaucoma surgery 159
   suspicious weak zonules 132
   uneven anterior chamber 191
   uveitis 96
   vitreous opacities 166
   weak zone 68-71, 74, 133
   wrinkle on anterior capsule 132
   wrinkling of face 193
Chamber depth, anterior 3
Convex anterior capsule 32
Corneal opacity 137, 140
Cortical cataract 40
   different variety of 84

D

Dense arcus senilis 192
Dense cataract with
   central corneal opacity 137
   hazy cornea 139
   inferior corneal opacity 139
   PSC 16
Dense nuclear cataract 124, 125
   with hazy cornea 125
   with shallow anterior chamber 124
Dense posterior subcapsular cataract 87
Developmental cataract, different variety of 77

Diffuse cataract 40, 56, 59, 60, 65, 87, 184
   with posterior synechiae 88
   with soft and small size nucleus 67
   with vitreous opacities 166
Dilated pupil 24, 32, 34, 40, 81, 56, 98, 140, 177, 189

E

Ectropion uveae with hard cataract 101
Edema, corneal 159

F

Festoon shaped pupil 100
   with immature cataract 100
   with mature cataract 101
Foldable intraocular lens 13, 56, 77, 113, 132, 147
   implantation 166

G

Glaucoma filtration surgery 156

H

Hard cataract 38-40, 42, 53, 118, 119, 152, 153, 170, 189
Hard cataract with
   corneal opacity 140
   dilated pupil 39
   early pterygium 170
   floppy iris 151
   hazy cornea 42
   posterior synechiae 97
   PSC 41
   semidilated pupil 55
   shallow AC 48
   small pupil 46, 131
Hard nucleus with
   advanced pterygium 171
   diffuse cataract 45
   mature cataract 47
Hazy cornea 97, 119, 125, 138, 139, 153, 171, 180
Hypermature cataract 104, 106
Hypermature cataract with
   central corneal opacity 141f
   fibrotic anterior capsule 134
   inferior corneal opacity 141f
   inferior subluxation 103, 106
Hypermature hard cataract 105
   with inferior subluxation 104
Hypermature intumescent cataract 105
Hypermature milky cataract 105
Hypermature sclerotic cataract 104

I

Immature cataract 4, 52, 59, 81, 83, 84, 96, 100, 107, 108, 138, 145, 147, 152, 156, 157, 159, 170, 174, 183, 186, 190
Immature cataract with
   central dense nucleus 183
   floppy iris 152
   glaucoma 156
   minimal subluxation 106
   Mooren's ulcer 174
   peripheral corneal opacities 138
   posterior synechiae 96
   PSC 15
   pterygium 170
   small pupil 129
   subluxation 107
   superior subluxation 108
Intraocular lens implantation 130
Iris coloboma with
   dense cataract 162
   immature cataract 161
   soft cataract 163

L

Lens
   removal of 110
   subluxated 109
Leukoma
   adherent 191
   with cataract, adherent 192
   with posterior synechiae, adherent 93

M

Marfan syndrome 109
Mature cataract with
   corneal opacity 141f
   floppy iris 153
   hazy cornea 35
   liquefied cortex 32
   micro-ophthalmos 164
   posterior synechiae 99
   shallow anterior chamber 126
   small pupil 35
Microspherophakia 110

Mid-dilated pupil 58, 119, 124, 125, 159, 170, 184
Mooren's ulcer 174

N

Normal cataract 3, 4, 51

P

Peripheral corneal opacities 138
Peripheral iridotomy 157
Polar cataract, posterior 3, 18, 19, 21
Pseudoexfoliation cataract 127, 135
Pseudoexfoliation cataract with
    bulky nucleus 119
    shallow anterior chamber 126
    small pupil 116
    small size nucleus 116
Pseudoexfoliation with
    adequate size of nucleus 114
    black cataract 121
    cortical cataract 120
    hard cataract 118
    mature cataract 119
    soft cataract 117
    very hard cataract 121
Pseudoexfoliation, different variety of 114

S

Semidilated pupil 25, 57, 101, 117, 118, 187
Shallow anterior chamber 159, 165
Slit lamp examination 4-10, 12
Small cornea 164, 165
Small incision cataract surgery 103, 137, 163, 172, 175, 190
Small size nucleus 24, 52

Soft cataract with
    ASC and cortical cataract 27
    PSC and cortical cataract 27
    shallow anterior chamber 127
    small size nucleus 24
Soft cataract, Vitreous opacities with 167
Steroid-induced cataract 86
Subcapsular cataract with
    soft cataract 14
    subluxation 107
Subcapsular cataract
    posterior 3, 13, 14, 17, 19, 25, 59, 61, 68, 80, 86, 98, 100, 108, 179
    traumatic anterior 92
    traumatic diffuse anterior 92
Subluxation, inferior 104, 106

T

Traumatic cataract with
    iridodialysis 94
    localized iridodialysis 95
    rupture of anterior capsule 90

U

Undilated pupil 81

V

Very hard cataract 41, 44, 45, 48, 49, 121, 122, 134, 140, 189
    with brown and black color 44
    with calcified anterior capsule 49

Z

Zonular weakness 105